The Hormone & Bone Health 2-in-1 Collection

Science-Backed Nutrition, Recipes & Exercises to Balance Hormones, Strengthen Bones, Boost Energy & Restore Gut Health Naturally

Isabella Harmony

Reclaim Your Hormone Health

A Comprehensive Guide to Beat Adrenal Fatigue, Manage Weight, Balance Mood, Relieve Stress, Improve Sleep, and Support Gut Health for Lasting Vitality & Wellness

Isabella Harmony

Disclaimer Notice:

Please note that the information contained within this document is for educational purposes only. All effort has been executed to present accurate, up-to-date, and reliable, complete information. No warranties of any kind are declared or implied. Readers acknowledge that the author is not engaging in the rendering of legal, Financial, medical, or professional advice.

The content within this book has been derived from various sources. Please consult a licensed professional before attempting any techniques outlined in this book. By reading this document, the reader agrees that under no circumstances is the author responsible for any losses, direct or indirect, which are incurred as a result of the use of the information contained within this document, including but not limited to errors, omissions, or inaccuracies

A FREE Gift

To further support your journey, I've included five exclusive bonuses to help you get started and stay motivated:

1. **The 7-Day Hormone-Balancing Meal Plan**: Simplify your nutrition with easy-to-follow recipes designed to stabilize your hormones and boost your vitality.
2. **Hormone Health Tracker**: Gain insight into your daily habits by recording your energy levels, mood, sleep quality, and symptoms—an essential tool for recognizing patterns and progress.
3. **Stress-Relief Exercises Guide**: Reduce cortisol and find your calm with quick, effective techniques like breathing exercises, yoga stretches, and mindfulness tips.
4. **Quick Hormone Health Quiz**: This interactive quiz will help you identify potential hormonal imbalances and clarify where to focus your efforts.
5. **Essential Hormone Health Shopping List**: Save time with this curated list of foods and supplements that support hormonal balance and overall well-being.

Please on the link below of scan the QR code to access the bonuses.

https://kidssltessentials.com/reclaim-your-hormone-health/

Table of Contents

Reclaim Your Hormone Health

Thrive with Osteoporosis

Introduction

A few years ago, I found myself staring into the mirror, feeling like a stranger in my own body. Menopause had arrived with an intensity I wasn't prepared for. The unexpected weight gain, relentless gut issues, and sleepless nights left me searching for answers. I knew I couldn't be alone in this struggle, and that realization sparked a determination to find solutions—not just for myself, but for anyone facing similar challenges.

This book is the result of that journey. It's designed as a guide to help you navigate the complexities of hormone health. You'll find well-researched information and practical advice tailored to both men and women. Whether your goal is to manage adrenal fatigue, stabilize your mood, relieve stress, improve sleep, or support gut health, this book is your ally in achieving hormonal balance.

Check out the five bonuses I created for you on the gift page at the beginning of the book. These tools are designed to complement the chapters in this book and give you actionable steps to implement immediately. Be sure to make the most of these bonuses—they are here to empower you on your journey to hormonal health.

Hormonal health affects us all, making this book relevant whether you're experiencing current Toor focusing on prevention. Understanding how hormones influence your body empowers you to make informed choices at any life stage, from adolescence to older adulthood, supporting long-term health and vitality.

Interactive elements like self-assessments are included throughout the book to help you personalize your journey. Alongside well-grounded scientific research, you'll also find personal stories, creating a blend of information and relatability that makes the content engaging and practical.

Let me share a bit about myself. I've experienced firsthand the challenges of menopause, gut health issues, and insomnia. These personal struggles have driven my passion for uncovering and sharing solutions with others. My story, coupled with my research, forms the foundation of this book, offering guidance and reassurance as you embark on your own path to hormonal health.

This book is thoughtfully structured to guide you through the essentials of hormone health. It begins with a foundation of knowledge about hormones and their role in the body, followed by chapters addressing specific areas like adrenal fatigue, weight management, mood stability, stress relief, sleep improvement, and gut health. Each chapter builds on the last, creating a cohesive guide to help you take control of your health step by step. Here, you'll also discover the connection between hormonal health and osteoporosis, gaining insights into how hormones directly impact bone health. If this topic interests you, look out for my upcoming book, specifically on osteoporosis, which will dive even deeper into managing and preventing this condition.

I encourage you to engage with the material actively. This isn't just a book—it's a tool to empower you. Each section provides practical advice to incorporate into your daily life, guiding you toward lasting vitality and wellness.

As you begin this journey, it's important to set realistic expectations. The insights and strategies in this book can help you improve your energy, mood, weight, and overall well-being by achieving balanced hormones. While this journey requires patience and consistency, improved health and vitality rewards are well worth the effort.

Chapter 1: Understanding Hormonal Imbalances

One morning, I found myself staring at a lab report, puzzled by the numbers that seemed to narrate their own story. It was during my early experiences with menopause that I realized how little I understood about hormones, despite their profound impact on every facet of my life—from the quality of my sleep to the unpredictability of my mood. This chapter aims to unravel the complexities of hormones, the body's elusive chemical messengers. Understanding hormones is crucial if you've felt off-kilter without knowing why or are just curious about maintaining your health. Here, we explore their fundamental roles, how they function, and why they are integral to our well-being.

Hormones 101: The Body's Chemical Messengers

Hormones are pivotal to the body's numerous physiological processes. The endocrine glands produce these chemical messengers through the bloodstream to reach specific target cells and tissues. Once there, they bind to specialized receptors, triggering biological responses. Think of hormones as the body's communication system, relaying instructions for growth, metabolism, and even emotions. The endocrine system, comprising glands like the thyroid, pituitary, and adrenal, ensures timely and precise communications. For instance, the pancreas releases insulin, a peptide hormone, to regulate blood sugar levels, demonstrating a seamless interaction between endocrine function and metabolic control. This system's harmony is crucial for maintaining homeostasis, the body's balance and stability.

Hormones fall into several categories, each with distinct roles. Steroid hormones, such as cortisol and estrogen, are derived from cholesterol and directly permeate cell membranes to influence gene expression. Cortisol, often dubbed the stress hormone, helps manage your body's response to stress and maintains various functions, including blood pressure and metabolism. Estrogen plays a vital role in reproductive health and has implications for bone density and cardiovascular health. Peptide hormones, like insulin and growth hormone, consist of amino acids and typically act on surface cell receptors, initiating a series of intracellular events. Insulin regulates glucose uptake, crucial for energy production, while growth hormones stimulate growth and cell reproduction. Amine hormones, including adrenaline and thyroid hormones, derive from amino acids and are involved in immediate physiological responses. Adrenaline, released during stress, prepares the body for 'fight or flight' responses, whereas thyroid hormones are essential for regulating metabolism and energy levels.

The body maintains hormonal balance through intricate feedback mechanisms. Negative feedback loops resemble a thermostat system; signals are sent to reduce production when hormone levels reach a certain threshold. This feedback ensures that hormone levels remain within an optimal range, preventing excesses or deficiencies that can lead to disorders. A prime example is the hypothalamus-pituitary-adrenal (HPA) axis, a complex set of interactions among these three glands. When faced with stress, the hypothalamus prompts the pituitary gland to secrete ACTH, which stimulates the adrenal glands to produce cortisol. Once adequate cortisol levels are achieved, the hypothalamus receives a signal to taper production, thus maintaining equilibrium.

Real-world examples illuminate the pivotal roles of hormones in everyday life. Insulin, for instance, is crucial for blood sugar regulation. After you eat, insulin levels rise, facilitating glucose uptake by cells for energy. Without adequate insulin, as seen in diabetes, blood sugar levels can become dangerously high. Cortisol, on the other hand, exemplifies the body's stress response mediator. Whether you are meeting a tight deadline or facing a challenging situation, cortisol mobilizes energy reserves, sharpens focus, and adjusts immune responses. While this response is vital in the short term, chronic elevation can lead to adverse effects like weight gain and impaired immune function. Understanding these processes underscores the importance of hormonal balance for overall health and vitality.

Identifying Symptoms and Signals

As I delved deeper into understanding hormones, I realized the subtle yet profound ways they manifest in our daily lives. One of the most telling signs of hormonal imbalance is unexplained fatigue. Many of us find ourselves dragging through the day, even after a full night's rest, wondering why our energy levels have forsaken us. This pervasive tiredness can seep into every aspect of life, making simple tasks feel insurmountable. Coupled with this fatigue, mood swings and irritability often creep in, turning minor annoyances into significant grievances. These emotional upheavals can strain relationships and erode one's sense of well-being. For someone who has always been easygoing, the sudden shift to irritability can be both confusing and distressing. It's as if the body and mind are at odds, each pulling in different directions.

Daily life can become a juggling act when hormones are out of balance. Many people need help with weight management despite diligent efforts with diet and exercise. The scale refuses to budge, leaving them frustrated and questioning their approach. This seemingly unyielding weight gain can feel like a betrayal, especially when healthy habits are in place. Sleep, too, becomes a casualty. Irregular patterns often lead to daytime drowsiness, creating a cycle of exhaustion that is impossible to break. Imagine waking up tired, longing for the energy to tackle the day's demands, only to find yourself yawning through meetings or nodding off during evening activities. These disruptions are inconvenient and signal deeper imbalances that require attention.

Diagnosing hormonal imbalances involves both scientific and holistic approaches. Blood tests are a standard method, providing a glimpse into hormone levels and revealing potential irregularities. These tests can identify whether the thyroid is underactive, if cortisol levels are spiking at inappropriate times, or if insulin is behaving erratically. Alongside these tests, lifestyle assessments offer insights into possible contributing factors, such as stress levels, dietary habits, and exercise routines. Examining how these elements interact gives a clearer picture of one's hormonal health. It's crucial to remember that while these methods are informative, they only form part of the solution. A medical professional's guidance is invaluable when interpreting results and planning the best course of action.

Knowing when to seek help is vital. If symptoms persist despite lifestyle adjustments, it may be time to consult a healthcare provider. For instance, professional evaluation becomes necessary if fatigue remains despite adequate sleep and a balanced diet, or if mood swings continue to disrupt personal and work life. The impact of hormonal imbalances can significantly affect quality of life, making it essential to address them promptly. Early intervention can prevent more severe complications and lead to effective management strategies. Often, people wait too long, attributing these symptoms to stress or aging, when in reality, they could be the body's plea for help. Understanding and acting on these signals can lead to a more balanced and fulfilling life.

The Role of Hormones in Metabolism and Weight Regulation

Hormones are central players in the regulation of metabolism and weight. They influence how efficiently your body converts food into energy, stores fat, and manages hunger and satiety. A key player in this complex system is the thyroid gland, which produces hormones that regulate metabolic rate. Thyroid hormones act like the body's thermostat, increasing the metabolic rate. When thyroid hormone levels drop, metabolism slows, often leading to weight gain and feelings of lethargy. Conversely, an overactive thyroid can accelerate metabolism, causing weight loss and increased energy consumption. This delicate balance highlights the thyroid's significant role in maintaining metabolic harmony.

Insulin, produced by the pancreas, is another crucial hormone for metabolism, particularly in nutrient storage and energy utilization. Insulin facilitates the uptake of glucose into cells, ensuring that the body has a steady supply of energy. When insulin functions properly, it helps regulate blood sugar and store energy efficiently. However, insulin resistance can develop, especially in poor diet or sedentary lifestyle cases, leading to inefficient glucose uptake and increased fat storage. This condition often results in weight gain and poses a risk of developing type 2 diabetes. Understanding insulin's role underscores the importance of maintaining sensitivity to this hormone through healthy lifestyle choices.

Hormonal imbalances can profoundly impact weight management, often complicating efforts to maintain a healthy weight. Leptin and ghrelin, known as the "hunger hormones," play pivotal roles in regulating appetite. Leptin, produced by fat cells, signals the brain to reduce appetite when energy stores are sufficient. Ghrelin, on the other hand, stimulates hunger and is secreted primarily in the stomach. When these hormones are out of balance, feelings of hunger and fullness can become disrupted, leading to overeating or inadequate calorie intake. Moreover, cortisol, often associated with stress, can influence fat distribution, remarkably increasing abdominal fat storage when chronically elevated levels. This can occur even without excess caloric intake, highlighting the complex interplay between hormones and weight.

Several practical strategies can be employed to support metabolic health through hormonal balance. Nutritional choices play a significant role, particularly in supporting insulin sensitivity. A diet rich in whole foods, fiber, and healthy fats can enhance insulin function and stabilize blood sugar levels. Regular physical activity promotes hormone balance by improving metabolic rate and insulin sensitivity. A combination of aerobic exercises and strength training can be particularly effective. Stress management is equally important, as it helps regulate cortisol levels, reducing the risk of stress-related weight gain. Mindfulness practices, meditation, and adequate sleep can contribute to a more balanced hormonal environment.

Consider the story of Celia, who, despite following a low-calorie diet and exercising regularly, struggled with weight loss. After investigating further, she discovered that her cortisol levels were elevated due to chronic stress, contributing to her weight retention, particularly around the abdomen. By incorporating stress-reducing activities such as yoga and mindfulness into her routine, she was able to lower her cortisol levels and achieve weight loss. Her experience underscores the significant impact that hormonal balance can have on metabolism and weight regulation, offering hope and guidance to others facing similar challenges.

Stress and Its Impact on Hormonal Health

In the daily rush of modern life, stress often feels like an unavoidable companion. It creeps in, unbidden, affecting our mood, sleep, and health. Stress triggers a cascade of hormonal changes, the most notable being the release of cortisol. This hormone, produced by the adrenal glands, is pivotal in the body's stress response. The activation of the hypothalamus-pituitary-adrenal (HPA) axis marks the beginning of this process. In moments of acute stress—say, when you're about to give a presentation—cortisol levels spike, providing a burst of energy and increased alertness. This response is part of our survival mechanism, intended to help us face immediate threats. However, when stress becomes chronic, the constant elevation of cortisol can wreak havoc on the body, leading to a host of health issues.

Chronic stress manifests in various ways, often insidiously affecting hormonal health. You might notice increased fatigue, a feeling of exhaustion that no amount of sleep seems to alleviate. This burnout results from the body's relentless efforts to cope with prolonged stress. Mood disturbances, too, become more frequent, as chronic stress can disrupt neurotransmitter function, leading to anxiety or even depression. The emotional turbulence accompanying stress can make it challenging to maintain focus and enjoy daily activities. Over time, these symptoms not only affect your mental health but also contribute to physical ailments, creating a vicious cycle that can be difficult to break.

To mitigate the impact of stress on your hormones, it is crucial to adopt effective coping mechanisms. Mindfulness and relaxation techniques, such as meditation and deep breathing exercises, have proven beneficial in reducing stress levels and promoting hormonal balance. These practices anchor you in the present, helping to calm an overactive mind and soothe frayed nerves. Exercise is another powerful tool in stress management; it releases endorphins, which enhance mood, and helps regulate cortisol levels. Regular physical activity, whether it's a brisk walk in the park or a yoga session, can be a natural antidote to stress-induced hormonal imbalances.

Research supports the importance of managing stress for hormonal health. Studies have shown that chronic stress can lead to adrenal fatigue, a condition where the adrenal glands become overworked and produce insufficient hormones. This insufficiency can compound feelings of fatigue and malaise, making everyday tasks seem daunting. By implementing stress-reduction strategies, you can protect your adrenal health and maintain a more balanced hormonal environment. It's important to remember that stress is a part of life, but how you respond to it can make all the difference in preserving your well-being.

Sleep and Hormonal Balance

Sleep is a fundamental component of our lives, intricately intertwined with hormonal regulation. The body's internal clock, known as the circadian rhythm, orchestrates the sleep-wake cycle, which hinges largely on melatonin production. This hormone, secreted by the pineal gland, signals the body when it is time to sleep. As daylight fades, melatonin levels rise, nudging you toward rest. This process is essential for maintaining a healthy sleep pattern. Meanwhile, during the deeper stages of sleep, the pituitary gland releases growth hormone, which is crucial for tissue repair and muscle growth. These hormonal activities underscore the profound connection between sleep and overall well-being.

The consequences of sleep deprivation on hormonal health are far-reaching. When sleep is disrupted, cortisol, the stress hormone, often becomes imbalanced, leading to an altered rhythm that can persist throughout the day. This imbalance can leave you feeling perpetually stressed, even in calm situations. Furthermore, sleep deprivation affects the hormones leptin and ghrelin, which play significant roles in appetite regulation. Leptin, responsible for signaling fullness, decreases, while ghrelin, which stimulates hunger, increases. This imbalance can lead to weight gain, as you may find yourself reaching for snacks more frequently, even when you are not truly hungry.

Improving sleep hygiene is a practical step toward achieving hormonal balance. One effective strategy is to establish a consistent sleep schedule. Going to bed and waking up at the same time each day, even on weekends, helps regulate your body's clock. Additionally, creating a restful sleep environment can significantly enhance sleep quality. Consider reducing screen time before bed, as the blue light emitted by devices can interfere with melatonin production. Instead, engage in calming activities, such as reading or taking a warm bath, to signal your body that it is time to wind down. These simple changes can pave the way for more restorative sleep.

Real-life examples highlight the transformative power of quality sleep. Consider the case of James, who, after years of feeling sluggish and irritable, decided to prioritize sleep. By committing to a regular sleep schedule and minimizing distractions in the bedroom, he experienced a marked improvement in energy levels and mood. This change enabled him to engage more fully in daily activities and maintain a healthier weight. Such stories underscore the importance of sleep in achieving hormonal harmony and overall health.

Gut Health: The Unsung Hero of Hormonal Balance

The intricate relationship between gut health and hormonal balance is a fascinating and often overlooked aspect of well-being. At the heart of this connection lies the gut microbiota, a diverse community of microorganisms residing in our intestines. These tiny organisms play a crucial role in regulating hormones by aiding digestion and absorption of nutrients, which are essential for hormone production and function. The gut can be considered a bustling city, teeming with life and activity, where each microbe has a specific role that contributes to the overall harmony of the body. The gut-brain axis further exemplifies this symbiotic relationship, as the gut communicates with the brain through neural, hormonal, and immune pathways. This bidirectional communication influences digestion, metabolism, mood, and mental health, highlighting the gut's significant impact on our overall hormonal landscape.

Recognizing the signs of poor gut health can be pivotal in addressing hormonal imbalances. Digestive issues such as bloating, gas, and irregular bowel movements can signal that the gut is not functioning optimally. These symptoms may seem benign initially, but they can indicate more profound hormonal disruptions. Inflammation is another critical aspect, as chronic inflammation can disrupt hormone production and regulation, leading to a cascade of health issues. An inflamed gut can impair the absorption of nutrients required for hormone synthesis, creating a detrimental feedback loop. When the gut is compromised, the body often raises the alarm through various symptoms, including unexplained weight changes, fatigue, and skin issues. These manifestations serve as a reminder that gut health is not isolated but is intricately connected to hormonal balance and overall well-being.

Improving gut health requires a multifaceted approach, beginning with dietary and lifestyle changes. Probiotic-rich foods like yogurt and kefir can introduce beneficial bacteria into the gut, promoting a healthy microbiome. Prebiotics, found in foods such as garlic, onions, and bananas, provide nourishment for these beneficial bacteria, supporting their growth and activity. Reducing processed food intake is equally important, as processed foods often contain additives and preservatives that can harm the gut lining and disrupt microbial communities. Adopting a diet rich in whole foods, fiber, and healthy fats can foster a supportive environment for gut health. Additionally, regular physical activity and adequate hydration can enhance gut motility and function, further supporting hormonal health.

The research underscores the pivotal role of the gut in hormonal health. Studies have demonstrated that probiotics can positively influence hormone regulation by modulating the gut microbiota, which can impact the endocrine system. For instance, certain strains of probiotics have been shown to affect hormones related to stress and appetite control, offering potential benefits for mood stability and weight management. This growing body of evidence highlights the importance of nurturing gut health as a critical factor in maintaining hormonal balance. By prioritizing gut health, individuals can lay a foundation for overall wellness, addressing hormonal imbalances at their source.

The intricate connection between gut health and hormones is a testament to the body's remarkable interconnectedness. By fostering a healthy gut environment through mindful dietary choices and lifestyle practices, we can support digestion and the regulation of hormones that influence every aspect of our health. This holistic approach empowers us to actively participate in our well-being, recognizing the gut as a pivotal ally in achieving balanced hormones and vibrant health. As we continue to explore the depths of this connection, it becomes clear that nurturing our gut is not just a path to digestive health but a gateway to enduring vitality.

Chapter 2: Personalized Hormone Health Plans

Imagine standing in your kitchen, overwhelmed by the multitude of supplements, diets, and wellness tips that promise to fix your hormonal woes. It can feel like trying to navigate a maze without a map. But what if the key to understanding your body lies within you and not in the myriad of external solutions? This chapter is about taking a closer look at your own hormones through self-assessment. By recognizing the unique signals your body sends, you can create a personalized plan that aligns with your specific needs.

Identifying your individual hormone levels is crucial for personalized health planning because it provides insights into how your body functions on a cellular level. Hormones, as you know, are the body's chemical messengers, orchestrating a delicate balance that affects everything from your mood to your metabolism. Recognizing personal symptoms is the first step in understanding whether your hormones are in harmony or out of sync. Perhaps you've noticed changes in your energy levels, mood swings, or unexpected weight gain. These are not random occurrences but signals that your body is sending to alert you of potential imbalances. Lifestyle factors, such as diet, sleep, and stress, play a significant role in maintaining hormonal balance. By paying attention to both your body's signals and your lifestyle, you can begin to piece together the puzzle of your hormonal health.

To start this journey of self-discovery, accessible tools and methods for self-assessment can provide valuable insights. Symptom checklists are a simple yet effective way to track changes in your body and identify patterns that may indicate hormonal imbalances. These checklists can help you pinpoint symptoms related to specific hormones, such as fatigue linked to cortisol levels or mood changes associated with estrogen fluctuations. Home testing kits, which analyze hormone levels through saliva or urine samples, offer a more detailed look at your hormonal health. These kits allow you to measure hormones like cortisol, estrogen, and testosterone in the comfort of your own home. They are user-friendly and can provide a snapshot of your current hormonal status, helping you understand where imbalances may lie.

Once you have gathered data through self-assessment, interpreting the results is the next crucial step. Understanding what your self-assessment reveals about your hormone health involves categorizing symptoms based on hormone types. For example, if you experience persistent fatigue, it may indicate issues with adrenal hormones like cortisol. On the other hand, irregular menstrual cycles could point to imbalances in reproductive hormones such as estrogen or progesterone. By categorizing symptoms, you can begin to see patterns and identify which hormones may be contributing to your current state of health. This understanding is the foundation for developing a personalized health plan tailored to your unique needs.

While self-assessment is a powerful tool, it is essential to know when to seek professional evaluation to confirm findings and gain a comprehensive understanding of your hormonal health. If your self-assessment indicates significant imbalances or if symptoms persist despite lifestyle changes, consulting with a healthcare provider is advisable. A referral to an endocrinologist for specialized testing can provide a deeper insight into your hormonal profile. These professionals can conduct thorough evaluations using blood tests, saliva tests, and other diagnostic tools to assess hormone levels and identify underlying issues. Their expertise can guide you in developing an effective treatment plan, ensuring that your journey toward hormonal balance is both informed and supported by medical insights.

Self-Assessment Checklist

- Do you experience frequent fatigue despite adequate rest?
- Have you noticed unexplained weight changes?
- Are mood swings disrupting your daily life?
- Do you have irregular menstrual cycles or changes in libido?
- Are you experiencing sleep disturbances or insomnia?

This simple checklist can help you identify potential hormonal imbalances. Use it to explore your symptoms and consider whether further assessment is necessary.

Tailoring Your Health Plan

In a world where health advice often comes in a one-size-fits-all package, the idea of a personalized health plan stands out as a beacon of hope. Generic advice might provide a broad framework, but it often falls short of addressing the unique nuances of our individual bodies. Hormonal responses can vary significantly from person to person, influenced by factors like genetics, lifestyle, and even the environment. This variability is why a tailored approach is not only more effective but also essential for long-term success. Personalized strategies consider your specific hormonal profile, allowing for adjustments that align closely with your body's needs. The benefits of personalizing your health plan extend beyond immediate results, fostering sustainable habits that promote well-being over the years.

Developing a personalized health plan starts with setting specific health goals. These goals should reflect what you want to achieve, whether it's increased energy, balanced mood, or weight management. Clear goals provide direction and motivation, serving as a benchmark to measure progress. Identifying lifestyle changes that align with your individual needs is the next step. This involves examining your current habits and determining which ones support your hormonal balance and which need modification. Perhaps incorporating more movement into your day or adjusting your sleep schedule to improve rest could make a significant difference. Tailoring these changes to your life ensures they are practical and sustainable, increasing the likelihood of success.

Your personal preferences and daily routines play a crucial role in shaping your health plan. For instance, choosing physical activities you genuinely enjoy, like dancing, hiking, or swimming, makes it easier to stay active consistently. The same principle applies to dietary changes; adapting these changes to fit cultural preferences and personal tastes ensures they become a natural part of your lifestyle rather than a burdensome chore. If you love Mediterranean cuisine, incorporating its principles of healthy fats and fresh produce could support your hormonal health while satisfying your palate. The goal is to create a plan that feels less like a regimen and more like a lifestyle that you embrace wholeheartedly.

To illustrate the power of personalization, consider the story of Mina, who struggled with persistent fatigue and weight gain. After identifying a sensitivity to high-intensity workouts, she shifted to gentler forms of exercise like yoga and walking. Simultaneously, she adjusted her diet to include more plant-based foods, which aligned with her personal values and dietary preferences. These changes, tailored to her specific needs, not only improved her energy levels but also led to gradual weight loss and enhanced overall well-being. This example highlights how personalization can transform a generic plan into one that truly works for you, addressing your unique challenges and goals.

Ultimately, personalizing your health plan is about listening to your body and honoring its signals. It's about finding the right balance between structure and flexibility, allowing room for adjustments as your needs evolve. By tailoring your approach to fit your life, you create a plan that supports not just your hormonal health but your overall quality of life.

Overcoming Fatigue

Fatigue has a way of creeping into your life, turning once vibrant days into endless battles with exhaustion. At the heart of this chronic fatigue often lies an intricate web of hormonal imbalances. Your adrenal glands, nestled atop your kidneys, play a pivotal role in energy regulation. They produce hormones like cortisol and adrenaline, which are crucial for maintaining alertness and managing stress. However, when your adrenal glands become overworked due to chronic stress or poor lifestyle habits, cortisol production can become erratic. This can lead to a state known as adrenal fatigue, where you feel worn out despite adequate rest. Similarly, thyroid hormones are key players in regulating your metabolic rate. An underactive thyroid, or hypothyroidism, can slow down your metabolism, leaving you feeling sluggish and perpetually tired. Understanding these hormonal contributors is the first step towards reclaiming your energy and vitality.

Addressing fatigue through lifestyle changes can significantly boost your energy levels. One of the most effective strategies is establishing consistent sleep routines. Your body thrives on regularity; going to bed and waking up at the same time each day helps regulate your internal clock, promoting restorative sleep. In addition to regular sleep patterns, making nutritional adjustments can provide the energy boost you need. A diet rich in whole foods, particularly those high in complex carbohydrates and healthy fats, supports steady energy levels throughout the day. Foods like oats, avocados, and nuts can be beneficial. Staying hydrated is equally important, as dehydration can exacerbate feelings of fatigue. By making these lifestyle modifications, you can create an environment that supports your body's natural energy production processes.

The role of stress management in energy restoration cannot be overstated. Chronic stress not only drains your energy reserves but also disrupts hormone production. Incorporating mindfulness practices into your daily routine can be a turning point. Mindfulness encourages you to focus on the present moment, reducing stress and its impact on your hormones. Simple mindfulness exercises, such as observing your breath or practicing gratitude, can help calm an overactive mind. Alongside mindfulness, relaxation techniques like deep breathing can further enhance your ability to manage stress. Deep breathing activates the parasympathetic nervous system, promoting relaxation and reducing cortisol levels. By prioritizing stress management, you can restore balance to your hormones and, in turn, your energy levels.

Success stories of fatigue management illustrate the transformative power of addressing hormonal balance. Consider the case of Jan, who struggled with persistent fatigue for years. Despite getting eight hours of sleep, she felt exhausted by midday. After a thorough evaluation, she discovered that her cortisol levels were elevated due to chronic stress. By incorporating daily mindfulness meditation and adjusting her diet to include more whole foods, she experienced a significant increase in energy. Her vitality returned, allowing her to engage more fully in her work and personal life. This story highlights the profound impact that targeted lifestyle changes can have on restoring energy through hormonal balance.

Addressing Unexplained Weight Gain

Unexplained weight gain can be frustrating, especially when you've been vigilant about your diet and exercise. At times, the culprit is hidden within your body's intricate hormonal system. Insulin resistance, for instance, is a significant player in weight accumulation. This condition occurs when your cells become less responsive to insulin, a hormone crucial for regulating blood sugar levels. When insulin isn't working effectively, your body struggles to use glucose for energy, leading to increased fat storage, particularly around the abdomen. Cortisol, the stress hormone, also influences weight by promoting the storage of visceral fat. High levels of cortisol, especially when stress is chronic, can lead your body to hold onto fat as a survival mechanism. This fat tends to accumulate in the abdominal area, which is more than just a cosmetic concern; it poses health risks like cardiovascular disease. Understanding these hormonal influences is essential to managing weight healthily and sustainably.

To manage weight through hormone balance, consider dietary changes that improve insulin sensitivity. Incorporating foods rich in fiber, such as whole grains, legumes, and vegetables, can help stabilize blood sugar levels. These foods slow down digestion, providing a steady release of glucose into the bloodstream, which can improve insulin function. Healthy fats, like those found in avocados, nuts, and olive oil, can also enhance insulin sensitivity. Furthermore, reducing the intake of refined sugars and processed foods can prevent insulin spikes, supporting a more balanced hormonal environment. Regular exercise is another powerful tool in managing weight hormonally. Physical activity helps regulate hormones related to metabolism and appetite. Engaging in a mix of aerobic exercises, like walking or cycling, and resistance training can promote muscle growth, which in turn enhances your metabolic rate. Exercise also aids in reducing stress, indirectly helping to manage cortisol levels.

The psychological impact of weight gain is an aspect that often goes overlooked. It can affect self-esteem and lead to feelings of frustration or inadequacy. You might find yourself avoiding social situations or feeling self-conscious in your clothing. Addressing these emotions is as important as the physical aspects of weight management. Building self-esteem through a positive body image involves recognizing your worth beyond physical appearance. Practice self-compassion and remind yourself that your journey towards health is unique. Celebrate small victories and focus on the progress you're making rather than on the weight itself. Engaging in activities that make you feel good, whether it's a favorite hobby or spending time with loved ones, can improve your mental outlook and reinforce a healthy relationship with your body.

Consider the story of Tony, who, after years of unexplained weight gain, discovered that his cortisol levels were consistently elevated due to his stressful job. By prioritizing stress management techniques such as yoga and meditation, he was able to lower his cortisol levels. Coupled with a diet rich in whole foods and a regular exercise routine, he gradually lost weight and felt more energized. Another example is of Basma, who struggled with insulin resistance but managed to improve her condition by adopting a low-glycemic diet and engaging in regular physical activity. These real-life examples illustrate how understanding and addressing hormonal imbalances can lead to successful weight management. By focusing on hormonal health, you can take control of your weight in a way that feels less like a battle and more like a holistic approach to well-being.

Managing Stress

Stress is an unavoidable part of life, but its impact on your hormonal health can be profound. When stress becomes chronic, it disrupts the body's delicate hormonal balance, leading to a cascade of issues that can exacerbate existing conditions. The hypothalamus-pituitary-adrenal (HPA) axis plays a crucial role in the body's response to stress. It regulates the release of cortisol, the primary stress hormone. Under normal circumstances, cortisol provides the energy boost needed to tackle immediate challenges. However, when the HPA axis becomes dysregulated due to prolonged stress, cortisol levels can remain elevated or fluctuate erratically. This dysregulation can affect other hormones, such as insulin, thyroid hormones, and sex hormones, leading to fatigue, weight gain, and mood swings. Recognizing the connection between stress and hormonal imbalances is the first step in mitigating its effects.

To combat stress and its impact on your hormones, incorporating stress reduction techniques is essential. Yoga and meditation are two practices that have stood the test of time, offering a holistic approach to managing stress. Yoga combines physical postures with breath control and meditation, promoting relaxation and reducing cortisol levels. It also enhances flexibility and strength, contributing to overall well-being. Meditation, on the other hand, focuses on calming the mind, encouraging a state of mindfulness that helps you detach from stressors. Even a few minutes of meditation daily can significantly lower stress levels, improving hormonal health. Time management strategies are equally important. By organizing your day and setting realistic goals, you can reduce the sense of being overwhelmed, which often fuels stress. Prioritizing tasks and allowing for breaks can prevent burnout, ensuring that stress does not take root.

A supportive environment plays a pivotal role in stress management. Building a community support system can provide the emotional and practical support needed to navigate life's challenges. Whether it's family, friends, or a support group, having people to lean on can alleviate stress and promote a sense of belonging. Engaging in social activities and sharing experiences with others can build connections that buffer against stress. Support networks can also provide accountability and encouragement, making it easier to stick to stress management practices. The importance of community cannot be overstated, as it offers a sanctuary where you can express concerns and receive guidance, reinforcing your resilience against stress.

The research underscores the significance of stress management in hormonal regulation. Studies have shown that effective stress reduction techniques can lead to improved hormonal health. For example, a study on yoga practitioners found that regular practice significantly reduced cortisol levels and improved mood. Another study highlighted the benefits of mindfulness meditation in reducing anxiety and stress, leading to better hormonal balance. These findings emphasize the need to integrate stress management into daily routines.

Enhancing Sleep Quality

Sleep is a cornerstone of hormonal health, with crucial processes like growth hormone release and circadian rhythm regulation occurring during rest. Insufficient sleep disrupts these processes, impacting mood, metabolism, and immunity. To improve sleep quality, start with a consistent bedtime routine, such as dimming lights, reading, or taking a warm bath. Reducing screen time before bed is also vital, as blue light interferes with melatonin production.

Natural remedies like valerian root and techniques such as progressive muscle relaxation can further aid sleep. These approaches promote relaxation, reduce tension, and support restorative rest. Real-life examples, from busy parents to stressed students, highlight how better sleep transforms energy, focus, and emotional stability.

Consistency is key—small, intentional changes lead to significant improvements in sleep and hormonal balance over time. Next, we'll explore how nutrition supports hormonal health, equipping you with practical dietary strategies for balance and vitality.

Chapter 3: Nutrition and Hormonal Balance

When your hormones are balanced, your body functions at its best. However, when imbalances occur, they can disrupt this equilibrium and lead to various health challenges. In this chapter, we'll explore how the foods you eat can play a crucial role in supporting hormonal balance and overall well-being. By understanding the connection between nutrition and hormone health, you'll gain practical tools to make informed dietary choices that promote stability and vitality. Take control of your health by leveraging the power of nutrition for optimal hormonal function.

The concept of food as a tool for hormonal regulation is both empowering and practical. Certain foods have properties that can positively impact hormone production and balance. Omega-3 fatty acids, for instance, are renowned for their anti-inflammatory properties. Found in fatty fish like salmon and sardines, these essential fats help reduce inflammation in the body, which can otherwise disrupt hormonal balance. By incorporating omega-3-rich foods into your diet, you can support your body's natural ability to maintain stable hormone levels. Similarly, phytoestrogens found in plant-based foods like soy, flaxseeds, and lentils mimic the effects of estrogen, providing a natural way to support hormonal balance. These plant compounds can be particularly beneficial for those experiencing hormonal fluctuations, such as during menopause, by gently modulating estrogen levels and alleviating symptoms.

A balanced intake of macronutrients—carbohydrates, proteins, and fats—is crucial for hormonal health. Each macronutrient plays a distinct role in supporting your body's functions. Healthy fats, such as those found in avocados, nuts, and olive oil, are vital for hormone synthesis. They provide the building blocks for hormone production, ensuring that your body has the resources it needs to maintain hormonal equilibrium. Meanwhile, proteins, composed of amino acids, influence hormones like insulin and glucagon, which regulate blood sugar levels. A diet rich in lean proteins, such as chicken, fish, and legumes, can help stabilize blood sugar and prevent insulin spikes, promoting energy balance and reducing the risk of insulin resistance. Carbohydrates, particularly those from whole grains and vegetables, provide the necessary energy to fuel your body's processes, supporting overall metabolic health.

Equally important are the micronutrients—vitamins and minerals—essential for optimal hormone function. Zinc, for example, plays a pivotal role in testosterone production, impacting everything from muscle mass to mood. Foods like pumpkin seeds, chickpeas, and beef are excellent sources of zinc, offering a natural way to support testosterone levels. Vitamin D, often called the "sunshine vitamin," is another critical nutrient for hormone regulation. It influences the production and activity of hormones such as insulin and thyroid hormones, which affect metabolism and energy levels. Ensuring adequate vitamin D intake, whether through sun exposure or foods like fortified dairy products and fatty fish, can enhance your body's ability to regulate these hormones effectively.

To adopt a hormone-friendly diet, focus on incorporating whole, unprocessed foods into your meals. These foods provide the nutrients your body needs without the additives and preservatives found in processed foods that can disrupt hormonal balance. Emphasizing fruits, vegetables, whole grains, and lean proteins creates a foundation for good health. Limiting refined sugars and trans fats is equally important, as these can lead to inflammation and hormonal dysfunction. By making conscious food choices, you empower yourself to take control of your hormonal health, supporting a body that functions harmoniously and efficiently.

Dietary Reflection Exercise

Consider keeping a food journal for one week. Note what you eat, how you feel afterwards, and any changes in your energy or mood. Reflect on whether certain foods correlate with feeling more balanced or experiencing symptoms like fatigue or mood swings. This exercise can provide insights into how your diet impacts your hormonal health, guiding you in making informed dietary adjustments.

Superfoods: Nature's Pharmacy

Superfoods have earned their title due to their dense nutrient content and the exceptional benefits they offer, particularly in supporting hormonal balance. These foods go beyond basic nutrition, providing compounds that can profoundly influence your body's hormonal health. Antioxidant-rich berries, such as blueberries and strawberries, are a prime example. These vibrant fruits are packed with vitamins, minerals, and antioxidants that combat oxidative stress, a factor known to disrupt hormone function. By reducing oxidative damage, these berries help maintain the cells' integrity in hormone production and regulation. Leafy greens, like kale and spinach, are another powerhouse. They offer a rich supply of vitamins A, C, and K and essential minerals like magnesium and calcium, which are crucial for various hormonal processes. Their high fiber content also supports gut health, indirectly influencing hormone balance by promoting efficient nutrient absorption.

Specific superfoods stand out for their hormone-supporting properties. Chia seeds, for instance, are small but mighty. They are an excellent source of omega-3 fatty acids, known for their anti-inflammatory effects, which play a vital role in maintaining hormonal equilibrium. These tiny seeds also provide fiber and protein, contributing to stable blood sugar levels and reducing insulin spikes. With their creamy texture and rich taste, avocados are another superfood worth including in your diet. They are abundant in healthy fats, particularly monounsaturated fats, which are essential for hormone synthesis. The fiber content in avocados further aids digestion and supports a healthy gut, both of which are important for hormone health.

Incorporating superfoods into your daily meals can be a delightful experience. Smoothies offer a versatile and easy way to consume these nutrient-dense foods. Consider blending spinach with flaxseed, chia seeds, and your favorite berries for a refreshing breakfast or snack. This combination not only tastes great but also packs a powerful nutritional punch. Alternatively, salads provide another avenue for incorporating superfoods into your diet. A hearty salad featuring kale and nuts, drizzled with olive oil and sprinkled with chia seeds, can serve as a satisfying meal that supports your hormonal health. These simple yet effective additions to your meals ensure that you receive the benefits of superfoods without overhauling your diet completely.

Research backs the efficacy of superfoods in promoting hormonal health. Turmeric, a vibrant yellow spice commonly used in curry dishes, has been extensively studied for its anti-inflammatory properties. Curcumin, the active compound in turmeric, has shown potential in reducing inflammation and modulating hormones, making it a valuable addition to a hormone-supportive diet. Studies have demonstrated that curcumin can influence cytokine production and reduce oxidative stress, both of which are important factors in maintaining hormonal balance. You can harness its benefits and support your body's natural hormone regulation processes by incorporating turmeric into your meals, whether in soups, teas, or as a seasoning for vegetables.

Superfood Integration Challenge

To explore the impact of superfoods on your hormone health, try incorporating at least two superfoods into your meals each day for a week. Track any mood, energy levels, or overall well-being changes in a journal. Reflect on how these foods may influence your health and consider continuing or expanding your use of superfoods based on your observations. This hands-on approach can provide personal insights into the power of superfoods in your diet.

Understanding Endocrine Disruptors

Every day, we unknowingly interact with substances that can meddle with our body's hormonal harmony—these are known as endocrine disruptors. Such substances are chemicals that can interfere with the normal functioning of your endocrine system, which is responsible for hormone production and regulation. They can mimic hormones, block their natural actions, or alter how hormones are produced, leading to potential bodily disruptions. Pesticides used in conventionally grown produce are a common source of these disruptors. By seeping into fruits and vegetables, they introduce chemicals that can mimic or obstruct hormones. Similarly, chemicals found in plastic containers, such as those used for food storage or packaging, can leach into food items, especially when heated, posing a risk to your hormonal balance.

You may not realize it, but everyday food items and packaging materials often harbor these hidden disruptors. One of the most notorious is Bisphenol A (BPA), commonly found in the lining of canned foods. BPA can seep into the food, especially if the cans are exposed to high temperatures or stored for long periods. Another group of disruptors is phthalates. These chemicals are present in plastic wraps and containers, and they have a tendency to leach into food, particularly when the plastic is heated, such as in microwaving. Phthalates can interfere with endocrine function, posing risks to your hormonal health. Regular exposure to these chemicals can gradually affect your body's hormonal equilibrium, leading to subtle yet significant health implications over time.

The implications of chronic exposure to endocrine disruptors can be profound and far-reaching. These chemicals have been linked to disruptions in reproductive hormones, potentially affecting fertility and leading to developmental issues. Over time, the interference caused by these disruptors can lead to increased risks of metabolic disorders, such as obesity and diabetes. They may also contribute to hormonal imbalances that can affect mood, energy levels, and overall health. The subtle impact of these substances often goes unnoticed until symptoms become pronounced, highlighting the importance of awareness and proactive measures to mitigate exposure.

To minimize your exposure to these harmful substances, consider incorporating practical strategies into your daily routine. Choosing organic produce is a simple yet effective step. Organic fruits and vegetables are grown without synthetic pesticides, reducing your exposure to these disruptors. Although organic options can be more expensive, prioritizing certain produce items, known as the "Dirty Dozen," can be a cost-effective approach. Additionally, using glass or stainless steel containers for food storage is a wise choice. Unlike plastic, these materials do not leach harmful chemicals into your food, even when exposed to heat. By making these minor adjustments, you can significantly reduce your contact with endocrine disruptors, supporting your body's natural hormonal functions.

Endocrine Disruptor Reduction Checklist

- Opt for organic produce, especially for items with high pesticide residues.
- Replace plastic food containers with glass or stainless steel alternatives.
- Avoid microwaving food in plastic containers or using plastic wrap.
- Be cautious with canned foods, looking for those labeled BPA-free.

- Stay informed about which everyday household items may contribute to endocrine disruption and seek safer alternatives.

By integrating these strategies into your lifestyle, you can take meaningful steps toward protecting your hormonal health and fostering a more balanced internal environment.

Meal Planning

Imagine your body's daily rhythm as a finely tuned dance, where each meal serves as a cue for the next step. Meal planning is not just about fulfilling dietary needs; it's a strategic approach to nurture hormonal balance. By structuring your meals, you create a consistent pattern that helps stabilize blood sugar levels, which is essential for maintaining hormonal harmony. Regular meal timing acts like a metronome, keeping your body's internal clock in sync. Sticking to regular meal times can help keep your blood sugar stable, reducing energy dips and cravings throughout the day. This stability supports insulin regulation, which is crucial for managing weight and energy levels.

A balanced distribution of macronutrients is at the heart of effective meal planning. Each meal should include a mindful blend of carbohydrates, proteins, and fats. This combination ensures that your body receives a steady supply of energy and essential nutrients. Including various food groups in your meals provides the diverse nutrients your body needs to function optimally. Think of your plate as a canvas, where colorful fruits and vegetables, lean proteins like chicken or tofu, and healthy fats like nuts or seeds come together to create a masterpiece of nutrition. Prioritizing nutrient-dense foods—those rich in vitamins, minerals, and antioxidants—can further enhance your body's ability to maintain hormonal balance. These foods not only nourish your body but also support cellular functions that are vital for hormone production.

Creating a meal plan doesn't have to be overwhelming. Start with simple, balanced meals that you can easily prepare and enjoy. Consider a bowl of oatmeal topped with a generous handful of nuts and berries for breakfast. This hearty combination provides complex carbohydrates and healthy fats, fueling your morning while keeping you satisfied. For lunch, a quinoa salad with grilled chicken and an array of colorful vegetables can offer the protein, fiber, and micronutrients your body craves. Such meals are delicious and strategically designed to support your hormonal health throughout the day.

Portion control plays a crucial role in maintaining hormone levels. It's not just about what you eat, but how much you eat. Large portions can lead to overeating, which may cause insulin spikes, eventually leading to insulin resistance, a condition that can disrupt your body's hormonal balance and contribute to weight gain. By being mindful of portion sizes and listening to your body's hunger cues, you can avoid these spikes and support your body's natural hormonal regulation. This approach helps maintain a steady energy supply, preventing the highs and lows that often lead to cravings and fatigue.

Adopting a structured meal plan tailored to your hormonal needs can transform how you feel and function. It's about making thoughtful choices that align with your body's natural rhythms and nutritional requirements. As you experiment with different foods and meal timings, pay attention to how your body responds. You might notice changes in your energy levels, mood, or even sleep patterns. These observations can guide you in refining your meal plan, ensuring that it supports your unique hormones. Whether preparing meals at home or making choices on the go, keeping these principles in mind can help you maintain hormonal stability and overall well-being.

Intermittent Fasting

Intermittent fasting has gained popularity as an approach for weight management and its potential benefits on hormonal health. This eating pattern involves cycling between eating and fasting periods, which can profoundly affect your body's hormonal balance. One of the most significant impacts of intermittent fasting is on insulin sensitivity. During fasting periods, your body's insulin levels drop significantly, making your cells more sensitive to insulin. This increased sensitivity can help regulate blood sugar levels and reduce the risk of insulin resistance, which can lead to type 2 diabetes. Additionally, intermittent fasting can influence growth hormone levels, a crucial hormone involved in muscle growth, fat metabolism, and overall vitality. Research suggests fasting can boost growth hormone production, supporting muscle maintenance and fat loss.

There are various methods of intermittent fasting, each with its unique approach. The 16/8 method is the most straightforward, involving a daily eating window of eight hours followed by a 16-hour fasting period. This method allows you to consume all your meals within a specific timeframe, such as between noon and 8 PM, giving your body a significant break from food intake. Another popular method is the 5:2 approach, which involves eating normally five days a week while restricting calorie intake to about 500-600 calories on two non-consecutive days. This pattern provides flexibility, allowing you to choose fasting days based on your schedule and lifestyle. Both methods balance feeding and fasting, offering a sustainable way to incorporate fasting into your routine.

When beginning intermittent fasting, it's essential to implement this lifestyle change safely and responsibly. Gradually adjusting to fasting periods can help your body adapt without the shock of sudden changes. Start by slowly increasing fasting periods over several weeks, allowing your body to become accustomed to the new eating pattern. Staying hydrated during fasting is also crucial; it helps maintain energy levels and supports bodily functions. Water, herbal teas, and black coffee can keep you hydrated without disrupting the fasting state. Listening to your body's signals is key; if you feel weak or dizzy, it may be necessary to adjust your approach or consult with a healthcare professional. These guidelines ensure that intermittent fasting becomes a supportive component of your health routine rather than a source of stress.

Scientific research supports the benefits of intermittent fasting for metabolic and hormonal health. Studies have demonstrated that fasting can improve metabolic markers, such as reduced blood sugar levels and lower triglycerides, which are beneficial for cardiovascular health. Furthermore, fasting has been shown to reduce oxidative stress and inflammation, both associated with aging and chronic diseases. By enhancing cellular repair processes and gene expression, intermittent fasting may offer protective benefits against certain diseases and promote longevity. These findings highlight the potential of intermittent fasting as a powerful tool for improving hormonal health, supporting your body's natural processes and enhancing overall well-being.

Gut-Boosting Foods

Your gut is more than just a place where digestion happens; it's a vital hub for hormone regulation, affecting everything from your energy levels to your mood. The gut microbiome, a complex community of trillions of microorganisms, plays a crucial role in hormone metabolism. These microorganisms aid in the breakdown of food, allowing essential nutrients to be absorbed and used in hormone production. A balanced gut microbiome supports synthesising and regulating hormones, including serotonin, often dubbed the "happiness hormone," which influences your emotional well-being. When the gut is healthy, it communicates effectively with the brain, helping to stabilize mood and reduce stress, creating a harmonious internal environment.

To promote gut health, consider incorporating foods that support its function. Fermented foods like kefir, sauerkraut, and miso are excellent choices. These foods are rich in probiotics—live bacteria that can help restore the balance of the gut microbiome. Kefir, for instance, is a fermented milk drink loaded with beneficial bacteria and yeast, which improve digestion and immune function. Sauerkraut, a tangy cabbage dish, is not only a great source of probiotics but also contains enzymes that aid in breaking down nutrients, enhancing their absorption. High-fiber foods such as beans, lentils, and whole grains also play a significant role in gut health. The fiber in these foods acts as a prebiotic, feeding the good bacteria in your gut and promoting a healthy microbiome.

Incorporating gut-friendly foods into your meals can be simple and enjoyable. Consider adding kimchi, a spicy fermented cabbage, to your stir-fries for an extra burst of flavor and probiotics. This Korean staple can transform a simple dish into a nutritious powerhouse. Including yogurt in your breakfast routine is another easy way to boost your gut health. Opt for natural, unsweetened yogurt with fresh fruits or a sprinkle of seeds for added nutrients. Yogurt is rich in probiotics, which can help maintain a balanced gut flora, supporting overall digestion and nutrient absorption. These small changes can significantly impact your gut health, making it easier for your body to regulate hormones effectively.

The benefits of maintaining a healthy gut extend beyond hormone regulation. A well-functioning gut enhances digestion, ensuring that your body efficiently extracts and utilizes nutrients from your food. This process is vital for overall health, providing the building blocks needed for various bodily functions. A healthy gut also plays a pivotal role in immune function. Approximately 70% of the immune system resides in the gut, making it a critical component of your body's defense mechanism. By supporting gut health, you bolster your immune system, helping to protect against infections and illnesses. The connection between gut health and overall well-being is profound, highlighting the importance of nurturing this often-overlooked aspect of health.

As we consider the profound impact of gut health on hormone regulation and overall well-being, it becomes clear that our dietary choices are powerful tools for maintaining balance. By incorporating foods that support gut function, you can foster an environment where your body thrives. This approach not only aids in hormone regulation but also contributes to a robust immune system and improved digestion. With these insights, you're well-equipped to make informed dietary choices that support your body's natural processes, paving the way for enhanced health and vitality.

In the next chapter, we will explore lifestyle modifications that can further support your hormonal health, providing practical strategies to integrate into your daily routine.

Chapter 4: Lifestyle Modifications for Hormonal Health

Imagine your body as a complex network where every system plays a vital role in keeping things running smoothly. Lifestyle changes act as helpful guides, steering you toward better hormonal health. By intentionally adjusting your daily habits, you can support your body's natural rhythms and create a sense of balance and vitality. This chapter focuses on practical steps to enhance your hormonal health and overall well-being.

Exercise and Hormone Regulation

Exercise is a cornerstone of hormonal health, acting as a powerful regulator of your body's internal systems. Different types of physical activity influence hormone production and balance in distinct ways. Aerobic exercise, such as brisk walking, jogging, or cycling, is crucial in reducing cortisol levels, the hormone often associated with stress. When cortisol remains elevated due to chronic stress, it can lead to weight gain, particularly around the abdomen, and interfere with sleep and mood. Incorporating regular aerobic exercise into your routine can help manage cortisol levels, reduce stress, and promote a sense of calm and well-being.

On the other hand, resistance training significantly impacts testosterone levels, a hormone vital for muscle growth, bone density, and energy levels. Whether through weightlifting, bodyweight exercises, or resistance bands, engaging in resistance training stimulates the release of testosterone, reduces stress, and promotes muscle development and enhances overall vitality. This type of exercise also promotes the release of growth hormones, aiding in tissue repair and recovery. By combining aerobic and resistance exercises, you create a balanced routine that supports multiple aspects of hormonal health, fostering resilience and strength in both body and mind.

The benefits of regular exercise on hormonal health extend beyond individual hormones. Consistent physical activity enhances insulin sensitivity, allowing your body to use glucose more effectively and reducing the risk of developing insulin resistance. This improvement in insulin function helps maintain stable blood sugar levels, preventing the energy crashes and cravings often associated with poor glucose regulation. Additionally, exercise stimulates the production of endorphins, the body's natural mood elevators. These chemicals interact with receptors in the brain to reduce pain perception and generate positive feelings, often referred to as the "runner's high." This endorphin boost can significantly improve your mood and emotional stability, contributing to a more positive outlook on life.

Creating a balanced exercise routine that maximizes hormonal benefits involves a thoughtful approach to structuring workouts. Aim to incorporate both cardio and strength training sessions throughout the week. For example, you may schedule aerobic activities like cycling or swimming on certain days and dedicate others to resistance exercises. Ensuring adequate recovery periods between workouts is important to allow your body to repair and adapt. Rest days are essential for preventing overtraining and maintaining hormonal balance. Listening to your body and adjusting your routine as needed can help you sustain an effective exercise regimen that supports your overall health.

Consider the story of Isla, who transformed her life through exercise. Struggling with low energy and mood swings, she committed to a regular workout routine, combining aerobic and resistance training. Over time, she experienced increased energy and greater emotional stability. Her story exemplifies the profound impact that exercise can have on hormonal health and overall well-being. By prioritizing physical activity, you can actively manage your hormones, paving the way for a healthier and more balanced life.

Exercise Reflection Exercise

Reflect on your current exercise routine and consider any changes you might make to enhance hormonal health. Are there new activities you'd like to try or an adjustment to your schedule that could improve balance? Consider keeping a journal to track your progress, noting any changes in energy, mood, or overall well-being. This reflection can guide you in creating an exercise plan that aligns with your health goals.

Mindfulness and Meditation

Imagine your mind as a bustling market filled with thoughts, plans, and worries competing for your attention. In such a crowded space, stress thrives, and with it, the hormone cortisol often runs rampant. Mindfulness offers a way to quiet the clamor, allowing you to focus on the present and reduce stress. This practice can be transformative for hormonal balance. By engaging in mindfulness, you activate the parasympathetic nervous system—the body's 'rest and digest' mode—which counteracts stress responses and lowers cortisol levels. This shift calms the mind and supports the body's natural ability to restore balance, fostering a sense of peace and well-being.

Various mindfulness and meditation techniques can be woven into your daily routine, each offering unique benefits. Guided meditation sessions, for example, provide structured guidance through calming exercises, helping you focus and relax. These sessions often involve visualization or concentration on the breath, making them ideal for beginners seeking an easy entry into meditation. Mindful breathing exercises, on the other hand, are simple yet effective for reducing stress. By focusing on the breath, you create a mental anchor, gently pulling your mind away from distractions and into a calm state. This practice can be done anywhere, whether you're at your desk or waiting in line, making it a versatile tool for stress management.

The physiological benefits of consistent mindfulness practice extend beyond stress reduction. Regular engagement in mindfulness enhances emotional regulation, allowing you to respond to life's challenges with greater calm and clarity. As you practice, you may find your reactions to stressors more measured, reducing the emotional rollercoaster that often accompanies hormonal imbalances. Moreover, mindfulness can improve focus and cognitive function. Training your mind to concentrate on the present moment enhances your ability to maintain attention on tasks, boosting productivity and reducing mental fatigue. These cognitive enhancements support daily functioning and contribute to long-term mental health.

Integrating mindfulness into your daily life can be a rewarding journey. Start by setting aside a dedicated time each day for practice, whether it's first thing in the morning or as a way to unwind before bed. Consistency is vital, as regular practice reinforces the benefits and helps establish mindfulness as a habit. Consider using apps like Headspace or Calm, which offer a variety of guided meditations and mindfulness exercises tailored to different needs and preferences. These tools provide structure and support, making incorporating mindfulness into your routine easier. You'll find what resonates with you as you explore different techniques, creating a personalized practice that supports your hormonal health and overall well-being.

Yoga: Poses and Practices

Yoga offers a unique blend of physical and mental benefits that can profoundly influence hormonal health. Through gentle movements and mindful breath control, yoga reduces stress, which is critical in maintaining hormonal balance. When you practice yoga, you engage in breath work that calms the nervous system, reducing the production of cortisol, the stress hormone. This calming effect extends beyond the mat, helping you manage daily stressors more easily. Additionally, yoga improves flexibility and strength, supporting your body's resilience and adaptability. By stretching and strengthening muscles, you enhance circulation and promote the efficient delivery of nutrients and oxygen, which are vital for hormonal regulation.

Certain yoga poses target specific glands, aiding in hormone regulation. The supported bridge pose, for instance, gently stimulates the thyroid gland, boosting its function. By opening the throat area, this pose encourages better thyroid health, which can lead to improved metabolism and energy levels. Another beneficial pose is the legs-up-the-wall pose, which aids in adrenal relaxation. This restorative pose allows the body to release tension and stress, giving the adrenal glands a much-needed break. By promoting relaxation, it helps regulate cortisol levels, contributing to a sense of calm and balance. These poses, among others, demonstrate yoga's capacity to support hormonal health through specific physical actions.

The influence of yoga on the endocrine system is profound. Regular practice can stimulate the pituitary gland, often referred to as the master gland, due to its role in regulating other hormonal glands. By engaging in poses that encourage inversion or gentle compression, you can enhance the pituitary's function, promoting overall hormonal harmony. Yoga also aids in regulating the adrenal glands, which are responsible for producing stress hormones. Through practices that emphasize relaxation and mindfulness, you can mitigate the effects of chronic stress, allowing the adrenal glands to function more effectively. This holistic approach underscores yoga's potential to support hormonal health, offering both physical and mental benefits.

To develop a consistent yoga practice, consider starting with accessible resources. Joining a local yoga class allows you to learn from experienced instructors who can guide you through poses safely. In-person classes also offer a sense of community, allowing you to connect with others on a similar path. Online yoga tutorials are a convenient alternative if attending a class isn't feasible. Many platforms offer classes tailored to various levels and needs, enabling you to practice at your own pace. By incorporating yoga into your routine, you create a space for self-care and balance, supporting your body's natural ability to regulate hormones.

The Impact of Sleep Hygiene

The Impact of Sleep Hygiene on Hormonal Health: A Form of Self-Care Sleep, often overlooked, is a fundamental form of self-care that underpins hormonal balance. Good sleep hygiene is more than just getting enough hours of rest; it's about the quality and consistency of your sleep patterns. Establishing a consistent sleep schedule is key. Going to bed and waking up at the same time each day helps regulate your body's internal clock, known as the circadian rhythm. This regularity supports the production of melatonin, the hormone that governs sleep-wake cycles and encourages restful sleep. A restful sleep environment is equally important. Consider the bedroom as a sanctuary, free from distractions like electronic devices and unnecessary light. A dark, cool, and quiet room can significantly enhance sleep quality, allowing your body to regulate its hormonal functions naturally.

Several habits can promote better sleep, starting with limiting caffeine intake in the afternoon. Caffeine is a stimulant that can linger in your system for hours, potentially disrupting your ability to fall asleep at night. Avoiding caffeine after lunch gives your body ample time to metabolize it, reducing its impact on your sleep. Establishing a bedtime routine is another effective strategy. This routine signals to your body that it is time to wind down. Activities such as reading, taking a warm bath, or practicing relaxation exercises can prepare your mind and body for sleep. Consistency in these practices can make it easier to fall asleep quickly and enjoy a more restful night.

The hormonal benefits of restful sleep are profound. When you sleep well, your body maintains balanced cortisol and melatonin levels. Cortisol, the stress hormone, follows a natural rhythm, peaking in the morning to help you wake up and gradually declining throughout the day. This decline is crucial for allowing melatonin to rise in the evening, signaling that it is time for sleep. Adequate sleep also supports the release of growth hormones, particularly during deep sleep. Growth hormones are vital in tissue repair, muscle growth, and overall health. By prioritizing quality sleep, you support these hormonal processes, promoting recovery and vitality.

Real-life examples illustrate the transformative power of improved sleep hygiene. Consider the case of Dev, who struggled with chronic stress and fatigue, constantly feeling drained despite getting enough hours of sleep. By implementing changes such as limiting screen time before bed and establishing a calming bedtime routine, he experienced a significant reduction in stress and an increase in energy levels. Another individual, Fatima found that by creating a more restful sleep environment—investing in blackout curtains and a comfortable mattress—she was able to fall asleep faster and wake up feeling refreshed. These stories demonstrate how simple adjustments can substantially improve sleep quality and, consequently, hormonal health.

Detoxifying Your Environment

In our daily lives, we are surrounded by an array of products and materials that, unbeknownst to us, may quietly undermine our hormonal health. Environmental detoxification isn't just a trendy buzzword; it's a practical approach to reducing exposure to harmful substances that can disrupt the delicate balance of your hormones. Endocrine disruptors, often found in everyday items, mimic or interfere with the body's natural hormones. These chemicals can alter the normal functioning of your endocrine system, leading to potential health issues over time. Identifying and minimizing these disruptors is crucial to creating a healthier living space. Your home should be a sanctuary that supports your well-being, free from pollutants that can compromise your health. By understanding the sources of these disruptors, you take the first step in reclaiming your living environment as a space of nourishment and safety.

Everyday household items frequently harbor endocrine disruptors, often without our awareness. Non-stick cookware, for instance, can release perfluoroalkyl substances (PFAS) when heated, interfering with hormone activity. These chemicals can seep into the food we prepare, entering our bodies without our notice. Similarly, synthetic fragrances in cleaning products, air fresheners, and personal care items often contain phthalates, which are linked to hormonal imbalances. These fragrances may make our homes smell pleasant, but they can introduce a chemical cocktail that affects your endocrine system. By being mindful of the products you bring into your home, you can reduce your exposure to these harmful substances, paving the way for a cleaner and healthier environment.

Detoxifying your environment involves practical and achievable steps. Opt for natural cleaning products made from plant-based ingredients instead of synthetic chemicals. These alternatives are effective and safer for your family and the planet. Choose glass or stainless steel over plastic in the kitchen for food storage and cooking. Unlike plastic, these materials do not leach harmful chemicals into your food, even when exposed to heat. Consider swapping out non-stick pans for those made of cast iron or stainless steel. These alternatives provide excellent cooking performance without the risk of chemical exposure. Making these changes gradually can lead to significant improvements in your environmental health.

The benefits of reducing exposure to toxins extend beyond just a cleaner home. Enhanced reproductive health is one of the most significant advantages. By minimizing contact with endocrine disruptors, you support your body's natural hormonal processes, which can lead to improved fertility and reproductive function. Additionally, reducing toxins can positively impact your energy levels and mood. Many people find that after detoxifying their environment, they experience a noticeable boost in vitality and emotional well-being. This transformation is not just about the physical benefits; it fosters a sense of empowerment, knowing that you are actively contributing to your health. A cleaner environment invites a sense of tranquility and clarity, allowing you to focus on what truly matters.

Environmental Detoxification Checklist

- Replace non-stick cookware with stainless steel or cast iron alternatives.
- Choose natural cleaning products that are free from synthetic fragrances and chemicals.
- Store food in glass or stainless steel containers to avoid plastic leaching.
- Use essential oils or natural air fresheners instead of synthetic options.
- Regularly ventilate your home to reduce indoor air pollutants.

Incorporating these changes into your lifestyle supports your body's ability to maintain hormonal balance and create a living space that fosters health and well-being.

Biohacking Your Lifestyle: Modern Techniques

In today's world, where technology seamlessly integrates with our daily lives, the concept of biohacking emerges as a compelling approach to optimizing health. Biohacking involves making informed lifestyle adjustments based on personal data, enabling you to tweak your body's performance and health outcomes. Imagine having the ability to understand your body's unique responses and make precise changes that align with your hormonal health goals. Wearable technology, like fitness trackers and smartwatches, plays a pivotal role in this process. These devices gather real-time data on your activity levels, heart rate, and even sleep patterns, providing insights into how your lifestyle choices impact your hormones. This data serves as a foundation for making targeted changes, allowing you to track progress and make informed decisions about your health.

Personalized nutrition plans are another facet of biohacking that can significantly impact hormonal balance. By understanding how different foods affect your body, you can tailor your diet to support optimal hormone production and regulation. Nutrigenomics, the study of how food interacts with your genes, offers insights into how individualized dietary choices can influence hormonal health. For example, some individuals may find that a diet rich in omega-3 fatty acids supports their hormonal balance, while others may benefit more from a diet emphasizing plant-based proteins. By experimenting with different foods and observing your body's response, you can create a nutrition plan that aligns with your unique hormonal needs.

Biohacking techniques offer innovative strategies for enhancing hormonal health. Cold exposure therapy, for example, involves brief exposure to cold temperatures to stimulate the production of beneficial hormones and improve metabolic function. This might include cold showers or cryotherapy sessions, which have been shown to increase endorphin levels and promote mental clarity. Additionally, cold exposure can enhance fat metabolism, supporting weight management and energy balance. Another technique uses nutrigenomics to inform dietary choices, allowing you to select foods that naturally boost hormone production and support metabolic health. By understanding the genetic factors that influence your response to food, you can make informed choices that optimize your diet for hormonal balance.

While biohacking offers numerous benefits, it also requires careful consideration and monitoring. The enhanced self-awareness that comes with tracking personal data can improve health outcomes as you gain insights into your body's unique rhythms and responses. However, biohacking has its challenges. It's essential to approach these techniques with a mindset of experimentation and adaptation. Only some strategies will work for some, and adjustments may be necessary to find what suits your body best. Careful monitoring is crucial to avoid potential pitfalls and ensure that changes support your overall health goals.

Starting a biohacking journey involves thoughtful planning and guidance. Consulting with healthcare professionals can provide valuable insights and help you safely navigate the complexities of biohacking. These experts can offer personalized advice based on your health history and goals, ensuring that your approach is both effective and safe. Keeping a detailed health and wellness journal is another valuable tool in your biohacking toolkit. You can identify patterns and make data-driven decisions about your health by recording changes in your diet, activity levels, and how you feel. This journal becomes a record of your progress, helping you refine your approach over time.

As you explore the potential of biohacking, remember that each step is an opportunity to learn more about your body and its needs. By embracing this mindset of curiosity and experimentation, you can unlock new levels of health and vitality. The journey is personal, and the insights gained can be transformative, empowering you to take control of your hormonal health and well-being.

Chapter 5: Natural Remedies and Supplements

Imagine walking through a vibrant garden, each plant holding secrets that can nurture your health. This vision reflects the essence of herbal remedies, which have been cherished for centuries for their ability to support hormonal balance. From ancient civilizations to modern-day practices, herbs have been revered for their therapeutic properties. In traditional medicine, plants like black cohosh and vitex were used to address women's health issues, while ashwagandha found a place in Ayurveda for its stress-relieving properties. These herbs were the original medicine, and their healing powers were passed down through generations. Today, as we seek alternatives to conventional treatments, these botanical allies offer a bridge between tradition and science.

The historical use of herbs in traditional medicine provides a rich tapestry of knowledge, illustrating how different cultures harnessed the power of plants to address health concerns. For instance, black cohosh has long been used by Native Americans to relieve menstrual discomfort and menopausal symptoms. Its efficacy is attributed to its ability to mimic the body's natural hormones, reducing hot flashes and mood swings. In modern pharmacology, black cohosh is recognized for its phytoestrogenic properties, offering a natural alternative to hormone replacement therapy. Similarly, vitex, or chaste tree, has been used since ancient Greece to regulate menstrual cycles and alleviate premenstrual syndrome. Its influence on the pituitary gland makes it a valuable tool in managing menstrual irregularities.

Ashwagandha, often called the "king of herbs," is renowned for its adaptogenic properties. It helps the body cope with stress by modulating cortisol levels. This herb has been a staple in Ayurvedic medicine, where it is used to enhance vitality and reduce anxiety. Modern studies support its efficacy, showing that ashwagandha can significantly lower cortisol levels, thereby reducing stress and improving overall well-being. Integrating these herbs into modern practice highlights a harmonious blend of ancient wisdom and contemporary science, offering holistic solutions for hormonal health.

Scientific research continues to validate the efficacy of herbal remedies, providing a robust foundation for their use in hormone health. Clinical trials on black cohosh have demonstrated its effectiveness in reducing menopausal symptoms, particularly hot flashes, which affect a significant number of women during menopause. These studies provide hope for those seeking relief without the risks associated with conventional hormone therapy. Ashwagandha's impact on cortisol levels has been studied extensively, with results showing significant reductions in stress-related symptoms and improvements in mood and energy. Such evidence underscores the potential of herbs to offer safe and effective alternatives for managing hormonal imbalances.

When considering herbal remedies, it is essential to incorporate them safely and effectively. Understanding the appropriate dosages and forms is crucial for maximizing their benefits while minimizing risks. Black cohosh is commonly available in capsule form, with recommended dosages typically ranging from 20 to 80 mg per day, depending on the specific product. Vitex can be found as a tincture or capsule, with a daily dosage of 20-40 mg often suggested for menstrual support. Ashwagandha is versatile, available as a powder, capsule, or tea, with dosages of around 300-600 mg daily being standard for stress relief. It is essential to consult with a healthcare provider, especially if you are taking other medications, as some herbs may interact with pharmaceuticals or exacerbate certain conditions.

Herbal Remedy Checklist

- **Black Cohosh**: Consider for menopausal symptoms such as hot flashes and mood swings. Commonly found in capsule form.
- **Vitex (Chaste Tree)**: Useful for menstrual irregularities and premenstrual syndrome. Available as tinctures and capsules.
- **Ashwagandha**: Ideal for managing stress-related hormonal imbalances. Offered in powders, capsules, and teas.

Incorporating these herbs into your wellness routine can offer a natural pathway to hormonal balance. Always prioritize safety by consulting with a healthcare professional and starting with recommended dosages. This approach ensures that you can enjoy the benefits of herbal remedies while minimizing potential risks.

Bioidentical Hormones

Bioidentical hormone therapy (BHT) offers a different approach to hormone replacement, one that aligns closely with the natural chemistry of your body. Unlike synthetic hormones, bioidentical hormones have a chemical structure identical to your body's hormones. This similarity can make them more compatible with your body's systems, potentially reducing unwanted side effects. Derived from plant sources such as soybeans and yams, bioidentical hormones are processed to create compounds that mimic the effects of natural hormones. They are available in various forms, including creams, gels, pills, and patches, providing flexibility and convenience in use. The ability to tailor these hormones to meet individual needs further distinguishes BHT from its synthetic counterparts.

The benefits of bioidentical hormones in hormone therapy are significant. One of the primary advantages is their potential for reduced side effects compared to synthetic hormones. Many people find that bioidentical hormones are more accessible for the body to assimilate, leading to fewer complications and a smoother transition during treatment. Moreover, BHT can be tailored to your specific hormonal requirements, allowing for a personalized approach to therapy. This customization means that the dosage can be adjusted based on your hormonal levels, lifestyle, and symptoms, offering a more targeted treatment. Such precision can enhance the effectiveness of the therapy, helping to achieve a better balance and improve the quality of life for those struggling with hormonal imbalances.

Despite the promising benefits, bioidentical hormones have their share of controversies and challenges. One of the main debates centers around the variability in manufacturing and potency. Because bioidentical hormones are often compounded in pharmacies, there can be inconsistencies in their production. This lack of standardization can lead to variations in hormone levels, which may affect their efficacy. Critics argue that with strict oversight, the quality and safety of compounded bioidentical hormones can be easier to guarantee. Additionally, the regulation of bioidentical hormones remains a contentious issue. While some healthcare professionals advocate for their use, others remain cautious due to the potential for uneven quality control and the absence of large-scale clinical trials comparing their long-term effects to those of synthetic hormones.

If you're considering pursuing BHT, it's crucial to do so under the guidance of a healthcare professional. Consulting with an endocrinologist or a hormone specialist can provide valuable insights into whether BHT suits you. These experts can conduct thorough evaluations, including blood tests, to assess your hormone levels accurately. Blood testing is often preferred over saliva tests for its precision, as it provides a comprehensive picture of your hormonal status. Once therapy begins, regular monitoring of hormone levels is essential to ensure optimal dosing and to make necessary adjustments. This ongoing assessment helps to maximize the benefits of BHT while minimizing potential risks, offering a path toward achieving hormonal balance.

Navigating the complexities of bioidentical hormone therapy can be challenging, but with the right support and information, it becomes a viable option for many seeking relief from hormonal imbalances. Understanding the nuances of BHT, from its chemical structure to its individualized application, empowers you to make informed decisions about your health. By working closely with healthcare providers, you can explore this natural approach to hormone therapy with confidence, knowing that it aligns with your body's needs and enhances your overall well-being.

Essential Supplements

The body is a complex system, with each part playing a critical role in maintaining overall health. Supplements are essential tools that support and guide these processes to keep everything in balance. Magnesium, for example, is crucial for reducing stress and supporting hormone production. It helps regulate cortisol, the hormone linked to stress, which can lead to reduced anxiety and improved sleep when kept in check. Additionally, magnesium supports healthy blood sugar levels by promoting insulin sensitivity, which lowers the risk of metabolic disorders. This combination of benefits makes magnesium a key player in maintaining hormonal balance and overall well-being.

Omega-3 fatty acids are another vital supplement known for their potent anti-inflammatory properties. These essential fats, abundant in fish oil, reduce inflammation that can disrupt hormonal balance. By modulating inflammatory pathways, omega-3s support overall health and mental well-being. They also play a role in brain health by supporting neurotransmitter function. This can improve mood regulation and cognitive function, making omega-3s a cornerstone of mental health support. Their benefits extend beyond the brain, aiding in regulating hormones associated with mood and stress, thereby creating a more stable emotional landscape.

Vitamin D, often called the "sunshine vitamin," is crucial for maintaining overall hormonal function. It acts as a regulator, influencing the production of hormones like insulin and those involved in calcium metabolism. Adequate vitamin D levels can support bone health by facilitating calcium absorption, reducing the risk of osteoporosis. Additionally, vitamin D has a role in the immune system, helping to protect against infections and inflammation. Its influence on hormone production means that a deficiency can lead to imbalances, affecting everything from energy levels to mood. Ensuring sufficient vitamin D intake is key to maintaining a well-functioning hormonal system.

Research supports the use of these supplements in promoting hormonal health. Studies have shown magnesium can significantly lower cortisol levels, relieving stress and enhancing sleep quality. Research on omega-3 fatty acids highlights their effectiveness in reducing symptoms of depression and anxiety, underscoring their role in mental health support. Vitamin D deficiency, on the other hand, has been linked to a variety of hormonal disorders, emphasizing the importance of maintaining adequate levels. These findings illustrate the profound impact that these supplements can have on your overall health and well-being.

Choosing the right supplements and using them effectively requires careful consideration. Recommended daily allowances can vary based on individual needs and health goals. A daily intake of 310-420 mg is generally advised for magnesium, depending on age and gender. Omega-3 fatty acids are often recommended at doses of 250-500 mg per day, focusing on EPA and DHA content. Vitamin D intake can vary widely, with 600-800 IU being a common recommendation, though higher doses may be necessary for those with deficiencies. Selecting high-quality supplements is equally important; look for products that have undergone third-party testing and are free from unnecessary additives. This ensures you receive the full benefits without compromising safety or efficacy.

Understanding the role of these supplements can empower you to make informed decisions about your health. Incorporating magnesium, omega-3s, and vitamin D into your wellness routine can support your body's natural processes and promote hormonal balance. These supplements offer a proactive approach to health, enhancing your ability to manage stress, maintain mental clarity, and support your overall well-being. Whether you're dealing with specific hormonal issues or seeking to improve your general health, these supplements provide valuable support in your journey towards balance and vitality.

The Role of Adaptogens in Stress

Adaptogens are like nature's answer to stress, offering a gentle yet powerful way to help the body find balance in times of turmoil. These natural substances enhance your body's ability to adapt to physical and emotional stressors by supporting the adrenal glands and their hormones. Think of them as your body's allies in maintaining homeostasis, the state of equilibrium that keeps you feeling centered and resilient. Common adaptogens include rhodiola and ginseng, which have been used for centuries in traditional medicine to boost energy, improve mood, and support overall well-being. Rhodiola, known for its ability to combat fatigue, is often referred to as the "golden root" because of its revered status in herbal medicine. Ginseng, another well-known adaptogen, is celebrated for enhancing vitality and reducing stress, making it a staple in many wellness routines.

The benefits of adaptogens for hormonal health are significant. These botanical wonders work by modulating the body's response to stress, particularly by balancing cortisol levels. Cortisol, often called the "stress hormone," plays a crucial role in how your body responds to stress. When cortisol levels are too high or too low, it can lead to fatigue, mood swings, and even weight gain. Adaptogens help normalize these levels, promoting a sense of calm and equilibrium. By supporting adrenal function, adaptogens enhance energy and reduce fatigue, making it easier to face daily challenges. They do not act on a single organ or system but rather improve the body's overall resistance to stress, providing a more holistic approach to health. Regular use of adaptogens can lead to improved mental clarity, enhanced mood, and increased physical endurance, all of which contribute to a more balanced life.

Scientific evidence supports the efficacy of adaptogens, with numerous studies highlighting their benefits. Research on Rhodiola, for instance, has shown its effectiveness in reducing stress and combating fatigue. A study published in the journal "Phytomedicine" found that participants who took Rhodiola extract reported significantly improved fatigue levels and overall well-being compared to those who took a placebo. Similarly, studies on ginseng have demonstrated its positive impact on adrenal function and its ability to enhance cognitive performance. The adaptogenic properties of ginseng make it particularly valuable in managing stress-related hormonal imbalances, offering a natural way to boost energy and resilience. These findings validate the traditional use of adaptogens and underscore their potential as a natural solution for maintaining hormonal health.

Incorporating adaptogens into your daily life can be both simple and rewarding. These herbs are available in various forms, including supplements, teas, and powders, making them easy to add to your routine. When selecting adaptogen supplements, choose reputable brands that ensure quality and potency. Begin with a low dosage, gradually increasing as your body adjusts, and consider personalizing your intake based on your stress levels and lifestyle needs. For instance, rhodiola can be taken in the morning to support energy throughout the day, while ginseng might be more beneficial during intense mental or physical exertion. Teas infused with adaptogens offer a soothing ritual that promotes hormonal balance and provides a moment of relaxation in your day. Remember, while adaptogens are generally safe, it's always wise to consult with a healthcare provider, especially if you have underlying health conditions or are taking other medications.

Balancing Hormones with Essential Oils

Essential oils have gained a reputation for their potent effects, not only in aromatherapy but also in supporting hormonal balance. These concentrated plant extracts offer a natural way to influence your body and mind through scent and topical application. Lavender oil, for instance, is renowned for its ability to promote relaxation and alleviate stress. Its calming properties can be particularly beneficial when life's pressures begin to mount, providing a gentle nudge towards tranquility. Whether you're dealing with anxiety or need to unwind, lavender oil can be a soothing companion. On the other hand, Clary sage oil has carved out a niche in women's health. It is often used to support menstrual and menopausal health, offering relief from cramps and mood swings by promoting hormonal equilibrium. This makes it a valuable ally for those navigating hormonal changes.

Beyond lavender and clary sage, other essential oils are known for their hormone-supporting properties. Geranium oil stands out for its balancing effects, particularly in maintaining hormonal harmony. This floral oil is often used to regulate emotions and promote stability, making it a go-to choice for balancing both body and mind. Peppermint oil, with its invigorating scent, is another powerhouse. Known for boosting energy and enhancing focus, peppermint oil can be a refreshing aid when mental clarity and alertness are needed. Its stimulating effects can help clear the fog of fatigue and renew your sense of vitality, making it a versatile tool in your wellness arsenal.

Incorporating essential oils into your daily routine is both simple and rewarding. Aromatherapy, using diffusers, allows you to fill your space with the therapeutic scents of these oils, creating an atmosphere of calm or invigoration, depending on your needs. For those who prefer direct application, topical use with carrier oils is an effective method. Carrier oils like jojoba or almond oil help dilute essential oils, reducing the risk of skin irritation and enhancing absorption. Mix a few drops of your chosen essential oil with a carrier oil and apply it to pulse points or areas of tension. This method allows the oils to work their magic directly on your skin, providing targeted relief and benefits.

Both scientific research and personal anecdotes support the efficacy of essential oils. Studies on lavender oil, for example, have shown its significant calming effects, reducing anxiety and promoting better sleep. By influencing the nervous system, lavender oil can create a soothing environment conducive to relaxation and restorative rest. Personal stories further illustrate the benefits of essential oils, with many individuals reporting improved mood and relaxation after incorporating these oils into their routines. Alison shared how diffusing lavender oil in her bedroom helped her unwind after long days, transforming her nightly routine into a peaceful ritual. Alice found that using clary sage oil during her menstrual cycle alleviated cramping and improved her emotional balance, allowing her to navigate her month easily.

Choosing high-quality products from reputable sources is important for those interested in exploring essential oils. Not all oils are created equal, and purity can significantly impact their effectiveness. Look for oils that are 100% pure, without additives or synthetic fragrances, to ensure you receive the full benefits. As with any wellness practice, start slowly and observe how your body responds. Essential oils can be powerful allies in promoting hormonal health and overall well-being, offering a natural way to support balance and harmony.

Safety and Efficacy

Navigating the world of supplements can feel overwhelming, especially when faced with many options, each promising miraculous result. But when it comes to integrating supplements into your routine, understanding their safety is paramount. Supplements, while beneficial, can interact with medications you're already taking, potentially altering their effectiveness or increasing the risk of side effects. This interaction is particularly concerning with medications affecting blood clotting or those processed by the liver. Furthermore, the risk of overdosage is real. They are taking more than the recommended amount of certain supplements can lead to toxicity, impacting organs like the liver and kidneys. Contamination is another concern; without strict regulation, some supplements may contain harmful substances not listed on their labels. Being informed about these risks is the first step in making safe and effective choices.

To choose supplements wisely, consider several strategies that ensure quality and efficacy. Look for products that have undergone third-party testing and carry certifications from reputable organizations. These seals of approval indicate that the supplement has been independently verified for quality and purity. Additionally, take the time to read ingredient labels carefully. Purity is crucial; avoid products with unnecessary fillers or additives, which can dilute the effectiveness of the active ingredients. Check for any allergens or substances that you may be sensitive to. By focusing on transparency and quality, you can better trust that the supplement will do what it claims to do without unwanted surprises.

Despite the potential benefits, there are common pitfalls to watch out for in supplement use. Misleading marketing claims can lead you to believe that a supplement is a cure-all. Be wary of products that make exaggerated promises, such as rapid weight loss or instant energy boosts. These claims often need more scientific backing and can lead to disappointment or even harm. Another mistake is relying solely on supplements without making necessary lifestyle changes. Supplements are meant to complement a healthy lifestyle, not replace it. Supplements alone are likely to produce the desired outcomes with a balanced diet, regular exercise, and adequate sleep. They work best when integrated into a holistic approach to well-being.

Professional guidance is invaluable when incorporating supplements into your health regimen. Consulting with healthcare providers or nutritionists can provide personalized insights based on your health status and needs. These professionals can help you understand which supplements are appropriate for you and how they interact with your current medications or conditions. Regular monitoring of your health status while using supplements is also advisable. This monitoring can include periodic blood tests or health assessments to ensure the supplements work as intended and adjust dosages if necessary. Such oversight helps prevent potential complications and ensures your supplement regimen supports overall health goals.

As we close this chapter, remember that supplements can be a powerful tool in supporting your health, but they require careful consideration and informed choices. With the right approach, they can complement a healthy lifestyle and contribute to your well-being. In the next chapter, we will explore the intricate connection between emotional and mental health and how they intertwine with hormonal balance, offering further insights into achieving lasting vitality.

Chapter 6: Emotional and Mental Health

The mind and body are deeply interconnected, working together to maintain overall health and well-being. At the core of this connection are hormones—chemical messengers that regulate emotions, stress responses, and physical health. Achieving hormonal balance requires understanding this intricate relationship, as mental states significantly affect hormone production and regulation.

The physiological link between the mind and body is evident in how stress affects hormone levels, mainly through the production of cortisol. When you experience stress, your body activates the hypothalamus-pituitary-adrenal (HPA) axis, releasing cortisol from the adrenal glands. This hormone helps you manage stress by providing quick energy and heightened alertness. However, chronic stress can lead to persistently high cortisol levels, which may contribute to adrenal fatigue and disrupt other hormonal functions. Elevated cortisol can impair immune function, leaving you more susceptible to illness and affecting your body's ability to recover from stress (Source: Harvard Health). The impact of emotional well-being on hormones is profound, influencing your physical health and your ability to cope with life's challenges.

Psychological stress disrupts hormonal balance, impacting both physical and mental health. Chronic stress over activates the HPA axis, leading to adrenal fatigue, exhaustion, irritability, and poor stress management. This imbalance can cause anxiety, depression, sleep disturbances, and hormonal disruptions affecting mood, energy, and well-being.

Stress-induced anxiety can impair digestion, causing bloating, indigestion, or IBS, while depression can disrupt sleep hormones, leading to insomnia and fatigue. These cycles highlight the need to address mental and physical health together for hormonal balance.

Psychosomatic medicine explores how psychological factors influence physical health, focusing on holistic treatments. Research links stress-related illnesses like hypertension to emotional states, emphasizing integrated care. Case studies demonstrate how addressing the mind and body together can restore balance and improve health.

Reflective Exercise: Mind-Body Awareness

Take a few moments each day to reflect on how your emotions influence your physical well-being. Consider keeping a journal to track your emotional states and any corresponding physical symptoms you experience. Note patterns and identify triggers that may contribute to stress or hormonal imbalances. This practice of self-awareness can provide valuable insights into the mind-body connection and help you develop strategies to promote balance and well-being.

Managing Mood Swings

In the complex dance of hormones, mood swings often take center stage, influenced by various hormonal shifts. Estrogen, a key player in this dynamic, fluctuates significantly during menstrual cycles, impacting mood and emotional stability. During the luteal phase, for example, estrogen levels drop, potentially leading to irritability or sadness. This ebb and flow can make you feel like you're on an emotional roller coaster. Similarly, testosterone, often associated with masculinity, plays a crucial role in regulating mood in both men and women. Low levels of testosterone can lead to feelings of lethargy, irritability, and even depression, affecting your emotional resilience. Recognizing these hormonal influences is the first step to understanding why mood swings occur and finding ways to manage them effectively.

Stabilizing mood amidst these hormonal influences requires a multifaceted approach, beginning with nutrition. A balanced diet rich in omega-3 fatty acids, complex carbohydrates, and lean proteins can support neurotransmitter production and promote emotional stability. Omega-3s, found in fatty fish and walnuts, are particularly beneficial for brain health, enhancing mood-regulating neurotransmitters like serotonin. Regular physical activity also plays a vital role in mood stabilization. Exercise releases endorphins, the body's natural mood elevators, which can enhance your well-being and counteract stress's effects. Whether it's a brisk walk, a yoga session, or a dance class, incorporating movement into your daily routine can provide a natural, effective way to manage mood swings.

Lifestyle factors further influence your emotional health. Maintaining regular sleep patterns is crucial, as sleep disruptions can exacerbate mood swings and hinder your ability to cope with stress. Aim for a consistent sleep schedule, prioritizing quality rest to support hormonal balance. Beyond sleep, social support is a pillar of emotional well-being. Engaging with friends, family, or community groups provides a sense of connection and belonging, which can buffer against stress and emotional upheavals. Whether it's a weekly coffee date or a virtual chat, these interactions foster resilience and offer a space to express emotions, share experiences, and receive support.

Personal stories of overcoming emotional challenges offer valuable insights and inspiration. Consider Jane, who struggled with intense mood swings due to hormonal fluctuations. By adopting a nutrient-rich diet and committing to a regular exercise routine, she noticed a marked improvement in her emotional stability. Her experience highlights the transformative power of lifestyle changes in managing mood swings. Similarly, Tom found that connecting with a local support group gave him a sense of community and understanding, helping him navigate the emotional ups and downs more easily. These testimonials serve as reminders that while mood swings can be challenging, they can also be managed with thoughtful strategies and support systems in place.

The Role of Mental Health

The intricate dance between mental health and hormone regulation is a testament to the body's interconnectedness. Mental health significantly influences hormone production; conversely, hormones affect mental well-being. Depression, for instance, can have a profound impact on thyroid function. The thyroid gland, responsible for regulating metabolism, can become sluggish due to depressive states, leading to hypothyroidism. This condition often manifests as fatigue, weight gain, and mood disturbances, creating a feedback loop where depression exacerbates thyroid dysfunction, and the resulting hormonal imbalance worsens mental health. It's a delicate balance, where one aspect can tip the scales, impacting the other continuously. Similarly, anxiety can affect reproductive hormones, disrupting menstrual cycles and affecting fertility. Chronic anxiety may lead to elevated levels of cortisol, the stress hormone, which can interfere with the normal production of reproductive hormones like estrogen and progesterone. This disruption can lead to irregular periods, mood swings, and a host of other symptoms that further contribute to anxiety, creating a vicious cycle that can be challenging to break.

Addressing the impact of mental health on hormones necessitates targeted interventions. Cognitive-behavioral therapy (CBT) is one such strategy that has proven effective in reducing stress and its hormonal implications. CBT focuses on identifying and changing negative thought patterns, which can alleviate stress and anxiety, indirectly supporting hormonal balance. By reframing how you perceive and react to stressors, CBT can help reduce cortisol levels, promoting a more balanced hormonal environment. Mindfulness-based stress reduction (MBSR) programs are another effective approach, emphasizing the importance of present-moment awareness. These programs combine mindfulness meditation and gentle yoga to cultivate a state of calm and reduce stress. Regularly practicing mindfulness can influence your body's response to stress, lowering cortisol production and fostering a more harmonious hormonal state.

Incorporating mental health practices into daily routines can significantly enhance hormonal health. Journaling, for example, provides a safe space for emotional processing, allowing you to express and reflect on your feelings. This practice can help clarify thoughts and reduce mental clutter, decreasing stress and its hormonal effects. Art therapy, another valuable tool, offers a creative outlet for stress relief. Engaging in artistic activities, whether painting, drawing, or crafting, can help reduce anxiety and promote relaxation. These practices tap into the brain's natural reward systems, releasing endorphins and fostering a sense of well-being. By integrating such techniques into your daily life, you can support both your mental health and hormonal balance, creating a more resilient and adaptable state of being.

The research underscores the significant impact of mental health interventions on hormonal regulation. Studies have shown CBT can effectively lower stress hormone levels, highlighting its potential in promoting hormonal balance. A study examining the effects of CBT on cortisol levels in older adults with generalized anxiety disorder found that those who participated in CBT alongside medication experienced a significant reduction in cortisol levels compared to those who did not receive therapy. This finding illustrates the powerful role of mental health strategies in modulating hormonal responses, offering a pathway to improved well-being. Addressing the cognitive aspects of health can positively influence your hormonal environment, fostering overall wellness.

Stress Management Techniques

Managing stress is not just beneficial; it is crucial for maintaining both emotional and hormonal health. When stress strikes, your body produces cortisol and adrenaline, the hormones responsible for the "fight or flight" response. While these hormones are vital for short-term survival, their prolonged presence can lead to chronic stress-related disorders. These disorders may manifest as anxiety, depression, or even physical illnesses like hypertension. High levels of stress hormones can disrupt your body's balance, affecting everything from mood to immune function. By managing stress, you can reduce these hormonal spikes, promoting a more stable emotional state and preventing stress-related health issues.

Several techniques can help you effectively manage stress, each offering a unique approach to calming the mind and body. Progressive muscle relaxation is one such method, where you systematically tense and then release different muscle groups. This exercise helps you become more aware of physical tension and learn how to let it go, promoting relaxation. Guided imagery and visualization practices provide another pathway to stress reduction. By imagining peaceful scenes or situations, you engage your senses and induce a state of calm. These mental exercises can transport you to a place of tranquility, reducing anxiety and promoting a sense of well-being. Each method offers a different way to focus your mind, helping you to manage stress more effectively.

The benefits of regular stress management extend beyond immediate relief, improving both mental and physical health over time. By reducing stress, you can enhance your mood and emotional regulation, making it easier to navigate daily challenges gracefully. Stress management also bolsters immune function, increasing your resilience against illnesses. When your body is not constantly fighting stress, it can better focus on maintaining overall health and vitality. Your body's resilience improves, allowing you to recover quickly from setbacks.

Incorporating stress management into daily life doesn't have to be complex. Setting aside even a few minutes each day for relaxation can make a significant difference. Consider establishing a daily routine that includes a moment of calm, whether through meditation, deep breathing, or a simple walk in nature. Technology can also be a valuable ally in your stress management efforts. Stress management apps, such as Calm or Headspace, offer guided exercises and meditations that you can easily fit into your schedule. These tools make it easier to practice stress reduction consistently, helping you build the habit of relaxation into your daily life. By prioritizing stress management, you actively contribute to your emotional and hormonal health, creating a solid foundation for overall well-being.

Building Resilience: Psychological Strategies

Resilience can be seen as your psychological armor against the unpredictability of life, particularly when it comes to maintaining hormonal balance. It involves adaptive coping mechanisms and the ability to respond to stressors flexibly. Imagine resilience as a tree that bends with the wind rather than breaking. In hormonal health, resilience helps you manage stress more effectively, supporting hormonal balance and overall well-being. When you are resilient, you can better regulate stress hormones such as cortisol, minimizing their adverse effects on your body. This capacity is not just about bouncing back after challenges but also about growing stronger with each experience.

To build this resilience, consider adopting a growth mindset, which encourages viewing challenges as opportunities for learning rather than obstacles. Embrace the idea that your abilities and intelligence can be developed through dedication and hard work. This mindset fosters a love for learning and resilience, essential for great accomplishment. Practicing gratitude and positive thinking can also enhance your psychological resilience. By focusing on what you are grateful for, you shift your attention from negative to positive aspects of your life, which can reduce stress and improve your mood. This practice can be as simple as writing down three things you are grateful for each day. Over time, this habit can train your brain to recognize and appreciate the positive, supporting your mental and emotional health.

Resilience has a profound impact on hormone regulation. When you cultivate resilience, you are essentially preparing your body to handle stress more efficiently, reducing stress hormone levels like cortisol. This reduction can have a ripple effect, enhancing your body's ability to recover from emotional setbacks more quickly. With lower cortisol levels, your body can focus on maintaining balance among other hormones, supporting everything from mood stability to immune function. This hormonal harmony contributes to a sense of well-being and vitality, reinforcing the benefits of building resilience.

Consider incorporating specific resilience-building exercises into your routine. Resilience training workshops offer structured environments where you can learn strategies to enhance your resilience, guided by experts who can provide personalized feedback. These workshops can help you develop skills like problem-solving, emotional regulation, and effective communication, all of which contribute to resilience. Additionally, daily affirmations and reflection exercises can further support your resilience-building efforts. Begin each day with positive affirmations that reinforce your strengths and capabilities. Reflect on your experiences at the end of the day, considering what you learned and how you grew from challenges. These practices can solidify your resilience by embedding positive patterns of thinking and behavior into your daily life.

When you engage in these exercises, you are not merely reacting to life's challenges but proactively building a foundation of strength and flexibility. This proactive approach can fortify your mental and emotional health, creating a buffer against stress that supports hormonal balance. These changes can enhance your quality of life, allowing you to navigate life's ups and downs with confidence and ease.

Incorporating these strategies can transform how you experience stress and challenges. As you become more resilient, you may find that you are better equipped to handle whatever comes your way. This resilience supports your hormonal health and enriches your overall well-being, enabling you to live a more balanced and fulfilling life.

Managing Anxiety and Depression: Hormonal Insights

Understanding the hormonal underpinnings of anxiety and depression can illuminate pathways to improved mental health. At the core of mood regulation is serotonin, a neurotransmitter that significantly influences feelings of well-being and happiness. Serotonin levels can be affected by various hormonal changes, such as fluctuations in estrogen and testosterone, which may contribute to mood disorders. Low serotonin levels can manifest as anxiety, depression, and irritability, creating a persistent sense of unease. Cortisol, the stress hormone, also plays a crucial role in anxiety disorders. High cortisol levels, often a result of chronic stress, can heighten anxiety, creating a cycle that is difficult to break. This hormonal interplay highlights the importance of addressing both the mind and body when managing anxiety and depression.

To manage these conditions hormonally, consider nutritional support for neurotransmitter production. Incorporating foods rich in tryptophan, an amino acid precursor to serotonin, can be beneficial. Turkey, eggs, and nuts are excellent sources of tryptophan, and including these in your diet can support serotonin synthesis. Additionally, ensuring adequate intake of vitamins B6 and B12, found in leafy greens and lean meats, can enhance neurotransmitter production. Regular exercise is another powerful ally in managing anxiety and depression. Physical activity boosts endorphins and serotonin, lifts mood, and reduces stress. Whether it's a morning jog, evening yoga, or a dance class, finding an activity you enjoy can significantly affect your mental health.

While lifestyle changes are vital, medication and therapy often play a crucial role in treating anxiety and depression. Antidepressants, particularly selective serotonin reuptake inhibitors (SSRIs), can help balance serotonin levels, alleviating symptoms of depression. It's essential to monitor thyroid function when using antidepressants, as imbalances can affect medication efficacy and overall well-being. Psychotherapy, particularly cognitive-behavioral therapy (CBT), offers a space for emotional processing and skill-building. CBT helps identify and alter negative thought patterns, leading to healthier coping mechanisms. This therapeutic approach can address the root causes of anxiety and depression, supporting both mental and hormonal health.

Consider the story of Sarah, who battled with depression for years. Through a combination of exercise, a balanced diet rich in omega-3 fatty acids, and therapy, she experienced a significant improvement in her mood. Her journey underscores the power of integrating hormonal insights into mental health care. Another example is Leo, who found relief from anxiety through regular meditation and dietary changes that supported neurotransmitter production. These case studies illustrate the profound impact that a holistic approach can have on overcoming anxiety and depression. By addressing both the hormonal and emotional aspects, these individuals found a way to reclaim their mental health and improve their quality of life.

Exploring anxiety and depression through the lens of hormonal health offers a holistic perspective on mental well-being. Recognizing the intricate connections between hormones and emotions provides a roadmap for effective management. As you consider these insights, remember that the path to mental health is multifaceted, requiring a blend of nutritional, physical, and therapeutic strategies. This approach addresses symptoms and nurtures the underlying factors, paving the way for lasting change. With these tools, you can navigate the complexities of mental health with confidence and resilience.

Chapter 7: Hormonal Health Across Different Life Stages

Throughout the stages of life, our bodies undergo remarkable transformations, each bringing a unique set of hormonal changes. Hormonal health plays a vital role in shaping our overall well-being, influencing everything from energy levels to mood and physical health. In this chapter, we begin by exploring adolescence, a pivotal phase marked by dramatic hormonal shifts that shape physical development, emotional well-being, and identity. From there, we examine how these changes evolve across the lifespan, eventually leading to other significant transitions, such as menopause, and their broader impact on health and well-being.

Hormonal Health in Adolescents

Adolescence is a pivotal time, marked by significant hormonal changes that lay the groundwork for adult health and well-being. During this phase, the body undergoes puberty, a complex transformation driven by sex hormones like estrogen in girls and testosterone in boys. These hormones initiate and regulate the development of secondary sexual characteristics, growth spurts, and reproductive maturation. As these hormones surge, they trigger physical developments such as increased height, changes in body composition, and the onset of menstruation or spermatogenesis. Adolescents may find themselves trying to navigate these changes, which are often accompanied by a mix of excitement and anxiety. Understanding these shifts is crucial, as they can affect the body, mind, and emotions, setting the stage for the challenges and opportunities that adolescence brings.

The hormonal upheaval of adolescence often manifests in common challenges that can impact both physical appearance and emotional well-being. Acne is one of the most visible and distressing issues, resulting from increased oil production and clogged pores. This skin condition, though common, can affect self-esteem and confidence during a time when social acceptance is paramount. Alongside physical changes, emotional volatility is another hallmark of adolescence. Mood swings, irritability, and heightened sensitivity can make teenagers feel as though they are on an emotional rollercoaster. These mood changes stem from the hormonal shifts affecting neurotransmitters in the brain, which regulate emotions and mood. For many adolescents, this volatility can lead to clashes with peers or family, adding to the complexity of navigating this life stage.

Supporting hormonal health during adolescence requires a multifaceted approach that addresses both physical and emotional needs. A balanced diet rich in nutrients promotes overall health and can help manage some of the physical changes associated with puberty. Encouraging teenagers to consume a variety of fruits, vegetables, lean proteins, and whole grains provides the vitamins and minerals necessary for healthy growth and skin health. Foods rich in zinc and omega-3 fatty acids, such as nuts and fish, can also help mitigate acne and support emotional stability. Regular exercise is another key component, promoting physical fitness, reducing stress, and enhancing mood by releasing endorphins. Activities that teenagers enjoy, such as team sports, dancing, or hiking, can encourage them to stay active and maintain a healthy lifestyle.

Open communication is vital in helping adolescents navigate their hormonal changes. Creating an environment where teenagers feel comfortable discussing their feelings and concerns can foster understanding and resilience. Encouraging open dialogue about the physical and emotional changes they are experiencing helps normalize these shifts and reduces feelings of isolation. Parents and caregivers can play a supportive role by listening actively and providing reassurance that these changes are a normal part of growing up. Additionally, equipping teenagers with information about their bodies and the expected changes can empower them to manage their health proactively. Education about self-care, hygiene, and stress management can bolster their confidence and ability to handle the challenges of adolescence.

Educational resources for parents and teens can provide valuable guidance and support during this transitional period. Books and workshops focused on adolescent health can offer insights into the physical and emotional changes occurring during puberty. These resources can equip families with knowledge and strategies to support their teenagers' development. Online support communities also offer a platform for parents to connect, share experiences, and seek advice from others navigating similar challenges. These communities can provide reassurance and practical tips for managing the ups and downs of adolescence, fostering a sense of community and shared understanding.

By utilizing these resources, families can navigate the complexities of adolescence together, promoting a nurturing and supportive environment for teenagers as they transition into adulthood.

Andropause: Understanding Male Hormonal Changes

For men, andropause represents a significant, albeit often less discussed, phase of hormonal transition. Commonly referred to as male menopause, this condition is marked by a gradual decline in testosterone levels. Unlike the sudden drop in hormones experienced by women during menopause, andropause unfolds more slowly, often over several years. Testosterone, a key hormone responsible for male characteristics and functions, affects everything from muscle mass to mood. As levels of this hormone decrease, men may notice changes that impact both physical and emotional health. Energy levels can wane, leaving a sense of fatigue that lingers despite rest. Libido, once robust, might diminish, affecting intimacy and personal relationships. Mood changes, including irritability or depression, can emerge, challenging emotional stability. Understanding these shifts is crucial for maintaining quality of life during this transition.

The symptoms of andropause manifest in various ways, often subtly at first but becoming more pronounced over time. Physically, men may experience a decrease in muscle mass and strength. This can lead to a reduction in physical capability and endurance, making daily tasks seem more taxing. Concurrently, there might be an increase in body fat, particularly around the abdomen, contributing to changes in body composition that impact self-esteem. Emotionally, men may find themselves grappling with mood swings that feel foreign and difficult to manage. The emotional upheaval can lead to feelings of frustration or sadness, which may be compounded by the physical changes co-occurring. Recognizing these symptoms as part of the natural aging process can be the first step in addressing them effectively.

Addressing the symptoms of andropause requires a proactive approach. One management option is testosterone replacement therapy (TRT), which can help replenish hormone levels and alleviate some of the associated symptoms. However, it's essential to weigh the potential benefits against the risks, such as increased acne or cardiovascular issues, and to have open discussions with healthcare providers. Regular physical activity becomes increasingly important during this time.

Incorporating exercises that build strength, such as resistance training, can help counteract the decline in muscle mass and improve overall fitness. Cardio exercises like walking or cycling can support cardiovascular health and manage weight. These activities enhance physical health and provide mental benefits, reducing stress and boosting mood by releasing endorphins.

Lifestyle changes that support hormonal health are vital during andropause. Nutrition plays a crucial role in maintaining testosterone levels. A balanced diet rich in lean proteins, healthy fats, and whole grains can provide the nutrients needed to support hormone production. Foods high in zinc, such as pumpkin seeds and lean meats, can be particularly beneficial for testosterone synthesis. Additionally, managing stress is paramount for emotional stability. Meditation, deep breathing, or mindfulness can help reduce cortisol levels, which can otherwise interfere with testosterone production. Creating a routine that includes relaxation and self-care can mitigate stress and promote a sense of well-being. While simple, these lifestyle adjustments can profoundly impact mitigating the effects of andropause and maintaining a healthy, active life.

These strategies address the symptoms and empower men to take control of their health during this transitional phase. By understanding the changes that andropause brings and implementing supportive measures, men can confidently navigate this stage. It's about embracing a new chapter with the tools and knowledge to maintain vitality and well-being.

Hormonal Changes During Pregnancy and Postpartum

The period of pregnancy is a profound symphony of hormonal changes orchestrating the creation of new life. As soon as conception occurs, your body produces high levels of estrogen and progesterone. These hormones are pivotal in maintaining the pregnancy. Estrogen increases significantly and helps develop the baby, and enhances uterine growth and blood flow, which is crucial for nourishing the developing fetus. Progesterone plays its part by maintaining the uterine lining and preventing contractions early in pregnancy. Meanwhile, human chorionic gonadotropin (hCG) makes its presence known early on, being responsible for maintaining the corpus luteum, which is crucial in early gestation. These hormonal shifts are necessary, yet they can also bring about a range of physical and emotional changes that you may find challenging.

The hormonal fluctuations during pregnancy can have a profound impact on both your physical and emotional health. Morning sickness, often experienced during the first trimester, is one of the most common complaints. The heightened levels of hCG are believed to be a contributing factor, leading to nausea and sometimes vomiting. Fatigue is another frequent companion, as your body works tirelessly to support the growing life within. The emotional rollercoaster of pregnancy is also a well-documented phenomenon. As estrogen and progesterone levels rise, they can affect neurotransmitters in the brain, leading to mood swings. You might find yourself elated one moment and inexplicably tearful the next. These mood changes, while unsettling, are a normal part of the journey and reflect the intricate dance of hormones at play.

After childbirth, the body undergoes another significant hormonal shift as it transitions from pregnancy to postpartum. This time is marked by a rapid decrease in estrogen and progesterone levels, which can contribute to the emotional turbulence often experienced after delivery. Supporting lactation and breastfeeding becomes a priority for many new mothers. The hormone prolactin, which increases during pregnancy, continues to rise and stimulates milk production. Ensuring adequate nutrition and hydration can aid in maintaining a healthy milk supply. Additionally, it's crucial to address postpartum depression and anxiety, which can affect up to 15% of new mothers. These conditions are not a reflection of your ability as a parent but rather a response to the hormonal and life changes you are experiencing. Seeking support from healthcare professionals, counseling, and peer groups can provide the necessary tools to navigate these challenges.

The postpartum period is unique to every mother, but shared experiences can offer comfort and guidance. Consider the story of a Alia, a first-time mother who faced significant postpartum anxiety. Initially hesitant to seek help, she eventually joined a support group for new mothers. There, she found a community that understood her struggles and offered a safe space to share and heal. Through the support of the group and professional counseling, she was able to manage her anxiety effectively and enjoy her time with her newborn. This example highlights the importance of building a support network during this time. Connecting with others who understand your experiences can provide reassurance and practical advice, making the transition to motherhood a more supported and enriching experience.

The hormonal shifts during pregnancy and postpartum are profound, shaping both physical and emotional landscapes. The journey through these changes is deeply personal, yet the shared experiences and support can help ease the path. Embracing the help of others and seeking professional guidance can empower you to navigate this transformative period with resilience and strength, fostering a nurturing environment for both you and your newborn.

Navigating Menopause

Menopause is a defining moment in a woman's life, characterized by profound physiological changes. As you approach menopause, your body undergoes a gradual decline in the production of estrogen and progesterone, the hormones that have regulated your reproductive system for decades. This decline marks the end of menstrual cycles and the beginning of a new phase. However, it also impacts other bodily functions, such as bone density and cardiovascular health. Estrogen plays a crucial role in maintaining bone strength, and its reduction can increase the risk of osteoporosis—a condition where bones become fragile and more susceptible to fractures. Cardiovascular health may also be affected, as estrogen is believed to protect the heart and blood vessels. The depletion of this hormone can thus elevate the risk of heart disease, making it essential to monitor heart health during this transition.

The symptoms of menopause can vary widely, but many women experience common challenges. Hot flashes and night sweats are often the most recognizable, leading to discomfort and sleep disturbances. You might find yourself waking in the middle of the night, drenched and unable to return to sleep, which can compound feelings of fatigue and irritability. Mood changes are another hallmark of menopause, as hormonal fluctuations can influence neurotransmitter levels, impacting emotional balance and leading to anxiety or depression. Sleep disturbances further exacerbate these mood changes, creating a cycle that can be difficult to break. Understanding these symptoms can help you prepare and manage them more effectively, ensuring they don't overshadow the quality of life.

Addressing the discomforts of menopause requires a multifaceted approach. Hormone Replacement Therapy (HRT) is one option that can help alleviate symptoms by supplementing the body with estrogen and, in some cases, progesterone. HRT can reduce the frequency and intensity of hot flashes and night sweats, improve mood, and support bone density. However, it's essential to consider the potential risks and benefits with a healthcare provider, as HRT may not be suitable for everyone. Lifestyle changes are also instrumental in managing symptoms. Incorporating a diet rich in calcium and vitamin D can bolster bone health, while regular weight-bearing exercises like walking or yoga help maintain bone strength and flexibility. These activities can also enhance cardiovascular health and overall well-being.

Real-life experiences offer valuable insights into navigating menopause. Consider the story of Margo, a woman who found relief through lifestyle adjustments. She managed her symptoms more effectively by incorporating daily walks, yoga, and a diet focused on whole foods. Margo also joined a community support group, where she shared experiences and learned from others facing similar challenges. The camaraderie and shared knowledge provided emotional support and practical tips that made the journey less daunting. Community support groups can be a lifeline, offering a space to share stories, strategies, and encouragement. They remind us that while menopause is a personal experience, it is also a shared one, with collective wisdom and support available to make the transition smoother and more empowering.

Reflection Section: Navigating Menopause

Consider your own experience with menopause. What symptoms have you encountered, and how have they impacted your daily life? Reflect on the strategies you've tried and their effectiveness. Are there lifestyle changes you could adopt to improve your well-being? This reflection can guide your approach, helping you navigate menopause with a sense of agency and resilience.

Aging Gracefully: Hormonal Health Beyond Menopause

As we age, our bodies adapt to new rhythms, and hormonal changes become an integral part of this transition. Beyond menopause, the decline in estrogen, testosterone, and growth hormone levels affects bone density, metabolism, energy levels, and overall vitality. This hormonal shift increases the risk of osteoporosis, impacts cardiovascular health, and brings visible changes like reduced skin elasticity and hair thinning. Addressing these changes requires proactive care, including tailored nutrition, regular exercise, and mindfulness of overall well-being.

Nutritional needs become more specific as we age. Calcium and vitamin D are essential for bone strength, while protein helps preserve muscle mass. Foods rich in omega-3 fatty acids support cognitive function and reduce inflammation. A diet abundant in colorful fruits, vegetables, and whole grains provides the nutrients and antioxidants necessary for combating oxidative stress and promoting hormonal stability and staying hydrated and maintaining balanced eating habits further support overall health.

Physical activity is equally vital, benefiting both physical and hormonal health. Weight-bearing exercises and resistance training strengthen bones and muscles, while activities like swimming, yoga, and tai chi improve flexibility and cardiovascular health. Exercise also promotes the release of endorphins, enhancing mood, cognitive function, and resilience against stress.

Emotional and mental well-being are closely tied to hormonal changes and require intentional support. Engaging in social activities, learning new skills, and pursuing hobbies keeps the mind sharp and fosters a sense of purpose. Coping with emotional shifts and loss becomes easier with strong social connections and a positive outlook.

Success stories highlight the transformative power of staying active and connected. For instance, older adults who practice yoga, maintain a garden, or participate in volunteer activities often experience better health, higher energy levels, and greater fulfillment. Community programs that promote wellness, social interaction, and lifelong learning provide additional opportunities to thrive in later years.

By nurturing the body and mind through a balanced lifestyle, aging becomes an opportunity to embrace vitality and fulfillment. As we move forward, the next chapter explores integrative approaches to hormone health, bridging traditional wisdom and modern practices for holistic well-being.

Chapter 8: Integrative Approaches and Future Directions

Functional medicine provides a holistic approach to health, addressing the root causes of hormonal imbalances rather than simply masking symptoms. This approach examines the complex interactions of lifestyle, nutrition, and environment to create a personalized pathway tailored to your unique needs. Advanced diagnostic tools, such as blood, saliva, and urine tests, are used to provide detailed insights into your hormonal health. These assessments form the basis for a customized healthcare plan aimed at restoring balance and optimizing overall well-being.

The holistic nature of functional medicine stands out in its ability to integrate various aspects of health. This approach offers a more effective strategy for managing hormonal issues by emphasizing lifestyle, nutrition, and environment. Collaboration with multiple healthcare providers ensures that all facets of your health are considered, creating a supportive network that addresses physical symptoms and emotional and psychological well-being. Nutritional therapies play a key role, targeting specific hormonal imbalances with tailored dietary interventions. For example, incorporating foods rich in omega-3 fatty acids can help manage inflammation, often linked to hormonal dysregulation. Stress reduction techniques, such as mindfulness and meditation, are integral to treatment plans, supporting the body's natural ability to balance hormones.

Functional medicine practices extend beyond traditional methods, offering innovative solutions for hormone health. Nutritional therapies are designed to target specific hormonal imbalances, using food as a tool to support and regulate hormone production. A diet rich in whole, unprocessed foods provides the nutrients needed for optimal hormone function. Meanwhile, stress reduction techniques, such as yoga or tai chi, are employed to support emotional and physical balance. These practices promote relaxation and help mitigate the effects of chronic stress, which can significantly impact hormone levels. By integrating these elements, functional medicine provides a comprehensive approach to hormonal health, addressing both the causes and symptoms of imbalance.

Case studies offer a glimpse into the transformative potential of functional medicine. Consider the case of an individual managing thyroid disorder through functional interventions. By adopting a nutrient-dense diet and incorporating targeted supplements, they experienced significant improvements in energy levels and overall well-being. Another case involved a person suffering from adrenal fatigue. They restored hormonal balance and regained their vitality through stress management techniques and lifestyle modifications. These examples highlight the success of functional medicine in addressing hormone-related conditions, demonstrating its effectiveness in achieving lasting health improvements.

Reflection Section: Assessing Your Health

Take a moment to consider your own health. What areas of your life could benefit from a more integrated approach? Reflect on your current lifestyle, nutrition, and environment. Are there specific changes that could support your hormonal health? Consider how functional medicine principles might apply to your unique situation. This reflection can be the first step in creating a personalized plan that addresses your individual needs, guiding you toward a path of balanced well-being.

The Future of Hormone Health: Innovations and Research

In the vibrant field of hormone health, advancements in science and technology are paving the way for more personalized and effective management strategies. One of the most promising developments is the rise of personalized hormone therapies. These treatments are designed to cater to the unique hormonal landscape of each individual, tailoring interventions to specific needs rather than employing a one-size-fits-all approach. This personalization is made possible by breakthroughs in genetic testing, which allow for a deeper understanding of hormone-related conditions. Genetic testing can reveal predispositions to hormonal imbalances and provide insights into how your body might respond to certain therapies, leading to more targeted and effective treatments.

Ongoing research is shedding new light on the intricate interactions between the gut microbiome and hormones. Scientists are uncovering how the trillions of bacteria residing in our intestines influence hormone production and regulation. This research suggests that gut health may play a significant role in hormonal balance, impacting everything from stress levels to metabolic health. Additionally, studies on the long-term effects of bioidentical hormones provide valuable insights into their safety and efficacy. These hormones, which mimic the body's natural hormones, offer an alternative to traditional hormone replacement therapies. Understanding their long-term impact is crucial for developing safer, more effective treatments for conditions like menopause and andropause.

Technology is also transforming the landscape of hormone health management. Wearable devices like smartwatches and fitness trackers have evolved beyond simple step counters. They now offer real-time hormone-tracking capabilities, providing immediate feedback on your body's hormonal fluctuations. This real-time data can help you identify patterns and triggers, allowing for more informed decision-making about your health. Mobile apps complement these devices by offering personalized health management tools. These apps can track symptoms, suggest lifestyle modifications, and even connect you with healthcare professionals, creating a seamless and integrated approach to managing your hormone health.

Looking to the future, the potential of artificial intelligence (AI) in hormone research is particularly exciting. AI can analyze vast amounts of data quickly and accurately, identifying patterns and correlations that might elude human researchers. This could lead to significant breakthroughs in understanding hormone-related conditions and developing new treatments. Innovations in hormone delivery systems are also on the horizon. Researchers are exploring new methods for delivering hormones more effectively, such as transdermal patches and implants that release hormones steadily over time. These innovations promise to enhance the precision and effectiveness of hormone therapies, reducing side effects and improving patient outcomes.

As these advancements continue to unfold, they hold the potential to revolutionize the way we understand and manage hormone health. With personalized therapies, cutting-edge technologies, and groundbreaking research, the future of hormone health looks brighter and more promising than ever.

Creating a Support Network

Navigating the complexities of hormonal health can feel daunting, and while personal efforts are crucial, the power of community support cannot be understated. Imagine walking into a room where everyone shares a common understanding of your struggles—this is the essence of community support. Social connections are not just nice to have; they are vital for enhancing hormonal well-being. Emotional support from those who genuinely understand your challenges can alleviate feelings of isolation and provide comfort. Sharing experiences with others creates a sense of camaraderie that can lift spirits and offer practical insights. Community resources, such as educational workshops and seminars, serve as valuable platforms for learning and empowerment. They equip you with knowledge and tools to manage hormone-related issues more effectively, reinforcing that you are not alone in this journey.

Support groups and online communities are pivotal in providing valuable information and encouragement. In today's digital age, online forums allow individuals from around the world to connect and share their experiences with hormone health. These platforms offer a wealth of knowledge, fostering discussions that might reveal new perspectives or solutions. Local meetups, on the other hand, bring people together face-to-face, creating spaces for shared learning and support. These gatherings can be a lifeline, offering opportunities to discuss personal stories, challenges, and triumphs. Being part of a community where people face similar issues helps normalize your experiences and provides reassurance that others share your struggles. This collective wisdom can be a powerful motivator, encouraging you to seek solutions and support.

Building a personal support network requires intentional effort, but the rewards are significant. Start by engaging family and friends in your health goals. Open conversations about hormonal challenges can foster understanding and support from those closest to you. Their involvement in your journey can provide encouragement and accountability, making it easier to stay on track with your health objectives. Additionally, seek out local or virtual support groups aligning with your needs. Whether you join a group focused on menopause, thyroid issues, or weight management, connecting with others who share similar concerns can provide both knowledge and empathy. These networks offer the chance to exchange ideas and strategies, creating a sense of community that bolsters your resolve.

The impact of community support on hormone health is profound, as illustrated by numerous testimonials. Consider the story of Jane, who managed her weight more effectively after joining a local support group. The shared accountability and encouragement she received from group members motivated her to stick to her health plan, leading to significant weight loss and improved self-esteem. Similarly, Mark found relief from stress through involvement in an online community where members shared stress reduction techniques and personal coping strategies. The sense of connection and shared experience helped him manage his stress levels more effectively, improving his overall hormonal balance. These stories highlight the transformative potential of community support, demonstrating how collective encouragement and shared experiences can enhance individual health outcomes.

Tracking Your Progress: Tools and Techniques

Understanding the nuances of your hormonal health involves more than just awareness; it requires active monitoring. Tracking your hormone health progress allows you to identify patterns and triggers, offering insights into the ebbs and flows of your body's internal chemistry. By observing these fluctuations, you can pinpoint the factors that might be contributing to your symptoms, such as stress or diet. This awareness is crucial for measuring the effectiveness of any interventions you have undertaken, whether they involve lifestyle changes or medical treatments. By keeping a record, you gain clarity on what works for your body and what doesn't, enabling you to make informed decisions about your health management strategies.

In today's digital age, various tools are available to help you monitor your hormone health. Health apps designed for daily symptom tracking provide a user-friendly interface for recording daily changes. These apps can track everything from mood swings to sleep patterns, offering a comprehensive view of your health over time. Wearable devices have also become invaluable in this regard. Smartwatches and fitness trackers monitor activity levels and sleep quality, delivering real-time data that can inform your health choices. These technologies make it easier to see the connections between your daily habits and hormonal health, providing a clearer picture of how your lifestyle affects your body.

To effectively utilize these tracking tools, set realistic goals and milestones. Start by defining your goals, such as improved energy levels or more restful sleep. These goals will guide your tracking efforts and help you stay motivated. As you gather data, regularly review it with a healthcare professional. This collaboration ensures that you interpret the information correctly and can adjust your strategies as needed. Healthcare providers can offer valuable insights into how your symptoms align with hormonal changes, providing a more nuanced understanding of your health.

Success stories illustrate the power of tracking in hormone health management. Take, for example, Esther, who struggled with low energy despite making several lifestyle changes. Using an activity tracker, she noticed patterns in her energy levels that correlated with her sleep quality. Adjusting her sleep routine, she found her energy improving significantly. Betty used a health app to monitor mood swings, discovering that increased stress at work was a significant trigger. With this knowledge, she implemented stress management techniques, leading to a marked improvement in emotional stability.

Engaging with tracking tools can be a transformative experience. It empowers you to take control of your health, offering tangible evidence of the impact of your daily choices. As you record your symptoms and habits, you better understand your body's needs and responses. This process informs your current health decisions and provides a valuable resource for future reference. By embracing technology and consistently monitoring your progress, you lay the foundation for a more balanced and informed approach to hormonal health. Tracking becomes a dialogue with your body, revealing insights that can guide you toward well-being.

Empowering Yourself: Take Control

Focusing on hormonal health, self-empowerment is your strongest ally. Taking an active role in managing your hormones is crucial for achieving and maintaining balance. This journey begins with increasing your knowledge and understanding of how hormones operate within your body. Hormones influence everything from your mood to your metabolism, and the more you know, the better equipped you are to make informed decisions. This enhanced understanding leads to improved decision-making in your health management, allowing you to tailor your strategies to your unique needs and circumstances. By embracing this proactive stance, you not only become the expert on your own body but also gain the confidence to navigate the complexities of hormonal health with assurance.

To empower yourself on this path, consider strategies that place you at the center of your health narrative. Start by educating yourself about hormone health topics. This doesn't mean you need a medical degree, but rather a commitment to learning the basics of how your hormones function and the factors that influence them. Books, reputable websites, and health seminars are excellent resources. Engaging in proactive health practices is equally important. This includes regular exercise, a balanced diet, and stress management techniques, all supporting hormonal balance. By taking small, consistent steps, you build a foundation of habits that reinforce your health goals. These practices support your physical health and empower you mentally and emotionally, reinforcing your commitment to taking charge.

Education and information are powerful tools in this empowerment process. Accessing reliable health information sources allows you to sift through the vast array of advice and find what truly resonates with you. Participating in workshops and seminars further expands your knowledge and connects you with experts and peers who share similar interests. These events provide a platform for asking questions, gaining insights, and learning about the latest advancements in hormone health. Armed with accurate information, you can confidently make choices that align with your health goals, whether that means adjusting your diet, exploring new therapies, or consulting with healthcare providers. This knowledge-driven approach transforms uncertainty into clarity, empowering you to lead your health journey with purpose.

Personal empowerment stories bring these concepts to life, showcasing the transformative power of self-education and proactive management. Take, for instance, the story of Emily, who faced relentless fatigue and mood swings. By immersing herself in hormone health literature, she discovered the impact of stress on her cortisol levels. She regained her energy and emotional stability by implementing stress reduction techniques and dietary changes. Similarly, Seb struggled with weight gain despite regular exercise. His journey into understanding insulin resistance revealed dietary tweaks that helped him shed pounds and increase vitality. These anecdotes illustrate that overcoming hormonal challenges is within reach with determination and the right knowledge. Their stories serve as a reminder that taking charge of your hormone health isn't just empowering—it's transformative.

Bridging the Gap: Hormone Health and Osteoporosis Connection

The intricate relationship between hormone health and bone health is a topic that demands attention, especially as we age. Hormones, particularly estrogen, play a pivotal role in maintaining bone density. Estrogen acts as a protective agent, slowing bone breakdown and promoting new bone tissue formation. This hormone helps regulate the bone resorption and formation cycle, ensuring that bone remains robust. As women approach menopause, a significant drop in estrogen levels can lead to accelerated bone loss, increasing the risk of osteoporosis. This condition, characterized by porous and fragile bones, makes individuals more susceptible to fractures, even from minor falls or injuries. Understanding this connection is crucial for anyone looking to protect their bone health as they age.

Thyroid hormones also play a critical role in bone metabolism. These hormones help regulate the body's metabolism, including the rate at which bone is broken down and rebuilt. Hyperthyroidism, a condition where the thyroid is overactive, can lead to increased bone resorption. This means that bone is broken down faster than it is replaced, decreasing bone density. The consequence is an elevated risk of osteoporosis, similar to what is seen in post-menopausal women due to estrogen decline. Individuals with thyroid imbalances must closely monitor their bone health and take proactive steps to mitigate these risks.

Several practical strategies can be employed to support bone health through hormonal balance. Nutritional support is fundamental. A calcium and vitamin D diet is essential for maintaining strong bones. Calcium is a crucial building block of bone tissue, while vitamin D facilitates calcium absorption in the body. Foods like dairy products, leafy greens, and fortified cereals can help meet your calcium needs. Exposure to sunlight and consuming fatty fish and fortified foods can provide adequate vitamin D. Regular weight-bearing exercises, such as walking, jogging, and resistance training, are vital for stimulating bone formation and maintaining bone density. These activities apply stress to the bones, prompting them to rebuild and strengthen.

Research has shown that hormone replacement therapy (HRT) can be effective in maintaining bone density and reducing the risk of fractures in post-menopausal women. Studies indicate that HRT can help restore some of the bone-protective benefits of estrogen, mitigating the rapid bone loss associated with menopause. However, it is essential to consult with a healthcare provider to weigh the benefits and risks of HRT, as it may not be suitable for everyone. Case studies further highlight the importance of hormonal regulation in bone health. Individuals who have managed their thyroid levels effectively have shown improvements in bone density, underscoring the significance of maintaining hormonal balance.

Throughout this exploration of hormone health and its impact on bone integrity, it becomes clear that maintaining balance is not just about addressing one aspect of health but understanding how interconnected systems work together. As you consider the strategies discussed, remember the importance of a holistic approach to your well-being.

A Personal Note From the Author

Dear Reader,

If this book has touched your life, brought you hope, or given you practical tools to reclaim your health, I'd be deeply grateful if you'd share your experience with others. Writing these pages was a labor of love—born from my own struggles and the journeys of those I've helped. But your story matters just as much.

Why Your Review Matters:

- It helps others like you find these solutions when they need them most.
- It lets me know what resonated, so I can create even more valuable resources.
- It's a ripple effect—your words might give someone the courage to start healing.

If a single page made you feel seen, or an exercise gave you relief, would you take a moment to leave a kind review? Just a sentence or two from the heart makes all the difference.

With sincere thanks,
Isabella Harmony

Conclusion

As you reach the end of this journey through "Reclaim Your Hormone Health," it's an opportune moment to reflect on the wealth of knowledge we've explored together. Throughout this book, we have delved into the intricate world of hormones and their profound impact on your daily life—from how you sleep to how you manage stress and maintain your mood. Understanding these chemical messengers allows you to take significant steps toward achieving lasting vitality and wellness.

The importance of maintaining hormonal balance cannot be overstated. Hormones are the silent architects of your health, affecting every aspect of your well-being. When in harmony, they empower you to live with energy and resilience. As someone who has personally navigated the challenges of menopause and hormonal imbalances, I can attest to the transformation that comes with achieving balance. It's not just about addressing symptoms; it's about reclaiming your life.

A personalized approach to hormone health is crucial. No two individuals are alike, and your hormonal journey is unique to you. Tailoring your health plan to your specific needs and preferences ensures that you are treating symptoms and addressing the root causes of imbalance. By understanding your body's signals and working with healthcare professionals, you can create a plan that supports your individual journey.

Nutrition and lifestyle choices play pivotal roles in supporting hormonal balance. A diet rich in whole, unprocessed foods and regular physical activity lays the foundation for optimal hormonal health. These choices fuel your body with the nutrients it needs to function efficiently. They also help regulate weight, improve sleep, and enhance mood. Remember, small, consistent changes can lead to significant improvements over time.

Equally important is the connection between mental and emotional health and hormonal balance. Psychological well-being is not separate from physical health; they are intertwined. Managing stress, nurturing emotional resilience, and fostering a positive mindset are integral to maintaining hormonal harmony. Prioritizing mental health through practices like mindfulness and meditation can profoundly affect your overall well-being.

As we explored the hormonal changes across different life stages, from adolescence to menopause and beyond, it became evident that each stage carries its own set of challenges and opportunities. Understanding these phases allows you to anticipate changes and adapt your strategies accordingly. Awareness is key, whether it's supporting bone health post-menopause or managing the transitions of adolescence.

The future of hormone health lies in integrating traditional wisdom with modern innovations. Combining established practices with cutting-edge research and technology offers a comprehensive approach to managing hormonal health. This integrative perspective empowers you to harness the best of both worlds, ensuring you have access to the most effective tools and strategies available.

Key takeaways from this book include the significance of a balanced diet, regular exercise, stress management, and personalized health plans. These elements form the pillars of your hormonal health strategy. Yet, beyond these strategies lies the most important aspect: self-empowerment. You hold the power to shape your hormonal journey. By staying informed, seeking support, and taking proactive steps, you can confidently navigate your path.

Community engagement is another powerful tool. Connecting with others with similar experiences provides a sense of belonging and support. Whether through online forums, local groups, or workshops, these connections can offer encouragement, practical advice, and shared wisdom.

As you move forward, I encourage you to implement the strategies discussed in this book. Track your progress, celebrate your achievements, and remain open to adjusting your approach as needed. Your journey to hormonal balance is a personal one, but it is also enriched by the shared experiences of others.

Thank you for entrusting me with your time and attention. It has been an honor to share these insights with you. Remember, you are not alone on this journey. You can achieve the balance and vitality you seek with determination, knowledge, and support. Here's to a future filled with health, happiness, and well-being.

References

- *Endocrine System: What It Is, Function, Organs \u0026 Diseases* https://my.clevelandclinic.org/health/body/21201-endocrine-system

- *Everything You Should Know About Hormonal Imbalance* https://www.healthline.com/health/hormonal-imbalance

- *Chronic stress puts your health at risk* https://www.mayoclinic.org/healthy-lifestyle/stress-management/in-depth/stress/art-20046037

- *The impact of the gut microbiota on the reproductive and ...* https://pmc.ncbi.nlm.nih.gov/articles/PMC7971312/#:~:text=It%20is%20possible%20that%20gut,sex%20hormones%20modify%20microbial%20diversity.Recently%2C%20it%20was%20reported%20that,and%20low%2Dgrade%20chronic%20inflammation.

- *Hormone Imbalance And Hormone Level Testing* https://www.testing.com/hormone-imbalance-and-hormone-level-testing/

- *Personalised health plans, powered by hormone testing ...* https://future-woman.com/

- *Bone Health in Adrenal Disorders - PMC* https://pmc.ncbi.nlm.nih.gov/articles/PMC5874185/

- *How to balance hormones naturally: 11 ways* https://www.medicalnewstoday.com/articles/324031

- *Hormone balancing diet: 9 foods to prioritize* https://www.singlecare.com/blog/hormone-balancing-diet/

- *Endocrine-Disrupting Chemicals (EDCs)* https://www.endocrine.org/patient-engagement/endocrine-library/edcs#:~:text=EDCs%20can%20disrupt%20many%20different,%2C%20certain%20cancers%2C%20respiratory%20problems%2C

- *Intermittent Fasting: Benefits, How It Works, and More*
  https://www.healthline.com/nutrition/10-health-benefits-of-intermittent-fasting#:~:text=Additionally%2C%20intermittent%20fasting%20enhances%20hormone,to%20use%20fat%20for%20energy.

- *Modulation of bone remodeling by the gut microbiota*
  https://www.nature.com/articles/s41413-023-00264-x

- *Exercise and hormonal secretion - PMC*
  https://pmc.ncbi.nlm.nih.gov/articles/PMC2425585/

- *Mindfulness from meditation associated with lower stress ...*
  https://www.ucdavis.edu/news/mindfulness-meditation-associated-lower-stress-hormone#:~:text=At%20an%20individual%20level%2C%20there,showed%20a%20decrease%20in%20cortisol.

- *Yoga Sequence for a Hormonal Imbalance*
  https://www.yogajournal.com/lifestyle/health/womens-health/yoga-sequence-hormonal-imbalance/

- *Endocrine Disruptors*
- https://www.niehs.nih.gov/health/topics/agents/endocrine

- *A review of effective herbal medicines in controlling ...*
  https://pmc.ncbi.nlm.nih.gov/articles/PMC5783135/

- *Bioidentical Hormones vs Synthetic Hormones*
  https://trocarsupplies.com/blogs/news/bioidentical-hormones-vs-synthetic-hormones?srsltid=AfmBOorijaiLhzSzCmWlMLLMu0ktv_jhAvw3KwxgQtaazLuOrdt8nJRu

- *Best Vitamins for Hormone Balance*
  https://rootfunctionalmedicine.com/best-vitamins-hormone-balance

- *The Role of Adaptogens in Stress And Fatigue Management*
  https://fullscript.com/blog/adaptogens

- *The Mind-Body Connection: Hormones and Mental Health*
  https://northtexasvitality.com/the-mind-body-connection-hormones-and-mental-health/

- *Understanding the stress response*
  https://www.health.harvard.edu/staying-healthy/understanding-the-stress-response

- *Cognitive-behavioral therapy augmentation of SSRI ...*
  https://pubmed.ncbi.nlm.nih.gov/26881447/

- *Glucocorticoid hormone as regulator and readout of ...*
  https://www.sciencedirect.com/science/article/pii/S2352154624000901

- *Osteoporosis and Menopause*
- https://www.webmd.com/menopause/osteoporosis-menopause

- *The Effect of Testosterone on Men With Andropause - PMC*
  https://pmc.ncbi.nlm.nih.gov/articles/PMC4706985/

- *Postpartum depression - Symptoms and causes - Mayo Clinic*
  https://www.mayoclinic.org/diseases-conditions/postpartum-depression/symptoms-causes/syc-20376617#:~:text=After%20childbirth%2C%20a%20dramatic%20drop,Emotional%20issues.

- *Addressing Hormonal Imbalances in Adolescents*
  https://www.rupahealth.com/post/addressing-hormonal-imbalances-in-adolescents

- *Functional Approach to Hormonal Imbalance*
  https://forumhealth.com/blog/restoring-hormonal-balance-a-functional-and-integrative-medicine-approach-for-men-and-women/

- *Hormones for menopause are safe, study finds. ...*
  https://www.npr.org/sections/health-shots/2024/05/01/1248525256/hormones-menopause-hormone-therapy-hot-flashes

- *The Effect of Support Group Method on Quality of Life in ...*
  https://pmc.ncbi.nlm.nih.gov/articles/PMC3521890/

- *Osteoporosis Due to Hormone Imbalance: An Overview ...*
  https://pmc.ncbi.nlm.nih.gov/articles/PMC8836058/

Thrive with Osteoporosis

Your Guide to Prevent Fractures, Build Strength, Improve
Balance, Embrace Natural Remedies, and Practice Safe
Exercises for Lifelong Mobility

Isabella Harmony

Introduction

When my mom was diagnosed with osteoporosis, it was like being thrown off balance, like the entire floor was pulled out from under us. She was a pillar in our family, always lively and energetic. The diagnosis was made after a minor fall, which resulted in a fracture of the bone. I saw her suffer from pain, physical disability, and the stress that comes with the disability. It was not only heartbreaking, but it also became a turning point for the whole family. Her story motivated me to learn more about osteoporosis and how I could help her and other sufferers improve their quality of life.

This book is a result of that experience. My goal is to give you all the information you need on how to live with and effectively manage osteoporosis. We will explore all aspects of it, including the medical aspect of the disease, practical tips, natural remedies, and expert advice. I want to present authentic clinical information, emotions, and personal experiences that can help improve the quality of life daily.

Osteoporosis is indeed a complicated condition, but the first step towards managing it is knowing as much as possible about it. This book will help you understand the condition, who is most likely to be affected, and how it can be diagnosed. We will review the most recent research on traditional treatments and natural remedies and present a fair view of your choices.

This book is intended for anyone who is an adult with a diagnosis of osteoporosis, people who may be at risk of developing it, and caregivers who support them. Osteoporosis is not gender selective; it occurs in both men and women. My focus is to provide the most comprehensive guide possible for anyone who has to deal with this condition.

My motivation for writing this book stems from my mom's journey, but it's also driven by extensive research. I have invested my time and numerous hours in reading up-to-date studies and collecting data from around the world. I want to help you, not confuse you with too many medical terminologies. The information is easy to understand, and the emphasis is placed on recommended strategies that can be applied in everyday life.

Now, let's discuss what you will find in the chapters ahead. First, we will examine osteoporosis, how it impacts your bones, and who will most likely develop it. The next section will discuss today's medical treatment, including medications and surgical options. We will also take a look at dietary recommendations and provide recipes that are healthy as well as tasty. Physical activity is critical in osteoporosis prevention; we will guide you through safe exercises at home. We will also discuss measures to avoid falls, emotional well-being, and ways to stay updated with the latest research.

Some recommendations that can be drawn from this book include how to handle osteoporosis, how to avoid fractures, and how to enhance bone health through nutrition and physical exercises. You will also read tips on seeking emotional support from family and friends or hiring a professional to help you. The aim is to equip you with adequate knowledge and tools to lead an active life despite osteoporosis.

To ensure that the information provided in this book is as accurate and up-to-date as possible, I've conducted extensive customer research and read the most recent scientific studies. I hope that it will be of use to you and that you will be able to refer to it anytime you feel the need for some assistance. Osteoporosis affects your lifestyle in many ways but does not dictate how you should live. If you have the knowledge and the right tools, you can take control of your bone health and continue to lead an active lifestyle. I assure you that you are not alone on this journey.

Chapter 1: Understanding Osteoporosis

A few years ago, I watched my mom struggle with everyday tasks after being diagnosed with osteoporosis. A simple fall broke her wrist, and from then on, our lives were filled with doctor visits, medications, and the constant worry of her falling again. That experience inspired me to learn all I could about osteoporosis. This book is built on her strength and our journey together, and I hope to guide you through yours.

Osteoporosis is a condition that weakens bones, making them fragile and prone to fractures from even minor trauma. Imagine bones as solid structures, like buildings. In osteoporosis, this structure deteriorates, losing density and strength. Healthy bones have a dense, honeycomb-like pattern, while osteoporotic bones have larger spaces within the honeycomb, making them weaker and more prone to break.

Osteoporosis affects millions worldwide, predominantly older adults. The International Osteoporosis Foundation estimates around 200 million people have the condition globally, with about 10 million in the U.S. alone. An additional 44 million Americans are at risk due to low bone density. Women, particularly postmenopausal women, are more affected, though men can develop it too, especially as they age. The economic and social costs are vast, with billions spent on healthcare and the significant impact of fractures leading to long-term disability and loss of independence.

A key challenge with osteoporosis is that it often has no symptoms until a fracture occurs. Common sites for fractures are the hip, spine, and wrist. Hip fractures usually require surgery and can lead to long-term disability, while vertebral fractures can cause chronic pain and height loss. Though wrist fractures are less severe, they still hinder daily tasks. Over time, osteoporosis can result in chronic pain, limited mobility, reliance on caregivers, and even increasing mortality rates.

It's important to differentiate between osteoporosis and osteopenia. Osteopenia is a less severe condition where bone density is below average but not as low as osteoporosis. Think of it as a warning sign that bones are weakening. Without intervention, osteopenia can progress into osteoporosis.

Preventative Measures for Osteopenia:

- Eat a balanced diet rich in calcium and vitamin D.

- Engage in regular weight-bearing exercise.

- Avoid smoking and excessive alcohol consumption.

Understanding Osteoporosis

Understanding osteoporosis is crucial for managing it effectively. By recognizing its impact on bones and knowing the signs to watch for, you can take proactive steps to protect your bone health. In the following sections, we'll explore treatments, diet, exercise plans, and strategies to prevent falls and fractures, helping you lead an active life despite osteoporosis.

Bones may seem rigid, but they constantly undergo remodeling. Made of collagen and calcium phosphate, bones gain flexibility from collagen and strength from calcium phosphate. Think of collagen as steel bars and calcium phosphate as concrete, forming a sturdy structure that supports the body.

Bone remodeling involves two key cell types: osteoclasts (which break down old bone) and osteoblasts (which build new bone). The balance between these processes maintains bone density. When disrupted, bone density decreases, leading to osteoporosis.

Bone density refers to the amount of minerals in bone tissue. The higher the density, the stronger the bones. Bone density is typically measured using a DEXA scan, which compares your bone density to that of a young, healthy person. A low score indicates osteopenia or osteoporosis, helping guide treatment decisions.

Several factors influence bone density, including family history, hormonal changes, and nutrition. Estrogen protects bones, so bone loss accelerates after menopause. A diet rich in calcium and vitamin D and regular weight-bearing exercise promotes healthy bones. Smoking and excessive alcohol consumption harm bone health, and conditions like rheumatoid arthritis and diabetes can also lead to bone loss over time.

Osteoporosis develops gradually and is influenced by both uncontrollable and controllable risk factors. Age and gender are primary risks—women, especially postmenopausal women, are at higher risk due to hormonal changes. Men also experience bone density loss but at a slower rate. Family history plays a role, and hormonal imbalances can weaken bones.

Lifestyle factors like poor nutrition, lack of physical activity, smoking, and excessive alcohol consumption also increase osteoporosis risk. A diet low in calcium and vitamin D deprives bones of essential nutrients, while weight-bearing exercises help maintain bone strength. Diseases like rheumatoid arthritis and diabetes, along with medications such as corticosteroids, can negatively affect bone health.

To reduce risk, focus on proper nutrition, including calcium-rich foods like leafy greens and dairy, and ensure adequate vitamin D through sunlight, food, or supplements. Regularly engage in weight-bearing exercise and strength training. Quitting smoking and limiting alcohol can also improve bone health.

Regular screening for osteoporosis is recommended, especially for those over 50 or with risk factors. Early detection through bone density tests can guide prevention and treatment strategies to minimize fractures and bone loss.

Taking steps to address these risk factors, making lifestyle changes, and working closely with healthcare providers are crucial to maintaining bone health and preventing osteoporosis.

Osteoporosis in Men vs. Women

Osteoporosis affects both sexes but is more common in postmenopausal women due to hormonal changes. Estrogen plays a crucial role in maintaining bone density by inhibiting osteoclasts, the cells responsible for bone breakdown. As estrogen levels drop during menopause, bone loss accelerates. In men, testosterone supports bone health by promoting osteoblast function, the cells that build new bone. While men's testosterone levels decline with age (andropause), this process is slower than women's postmenopausal bone loss.

Fracture patterns also differ between genders. Women commonly experience fractures in the spine, hip, and wrist, while men are more likely to suffer from hip and spine fractures. Women lose bone density rapidly in the early postmenopausal years, whereas men experience a gradual decline.

Hormone Replacement Therapy (HRT) is often recommended for women to slow bone loss post-menopause, though it comes with risks and requires a doctor's supervision. Men may be prescribed testosterone replacement therapy if needed, but this also requires careful monitoring due to potential side effects.

Acknowledging these gender-specific differences is essential for developing effective treatment and prevention strategies, ensuring that men and women receive the care they need to maintain strong bones and an active lifestyle.

The Stages of Osteoporosis

Osteoporosis progresses in stages, with each phase presenting different signs and symptoms. Early recognition and treatment are key to managing the disease effectively.

1. **Osteopenia:** The first stage, characterized by mildly reduced bone density, is often symptomless and detected through bone density tests. Osteopenia signals the need for preventative measures, like increasing calcium and vitamin D intake and regular weight-bearing exercises, to slow further bone loss.
2. **Early Osteoporosis:** In this stage, bone density has declined further, but symptoms may still be absent. Many people discover they have osteoporosis after a minor fracture. Early intervention through medication and lifestyle changes can prevent progression.
3. **Advanced Osteoporosis:** In the final stage, bones are fragile and prone to fractures from minor stress, like bending or coughing. Symptoms include chronic pain, height loss, and kyphosis (hunched back), which significantly affect mobility and quality of life. Multifaceted treatment—including medications, physical therapy, and pain management—becomes essential.

Diagnosis involves measuring bone density using a DEXA scan. A T-score between -1.0 and -2.5 indicates osteopenia, while a score below -2.5 points to osteoporosis. Severe osteoporosis is diagnosed when this low score is paired with a history of fractures.

Treatment depends on the stage of the disease. In osteopenia, lifestyle modifications can prevent further bone loss. Early osteoporosis is managed with medications like bisphosphonates or SERMs to preserve bone density and reduce fracture risk. In advanced stages, treatment focuses on medications, physical therapy, fall prevention, and in some cases, surgery to repair fractures.

Understanding these stages and their associated symptoms allows for better management of osteoporosis and helps in implementing timely interventions to maintain bone health and quality of life.

Living with osteoporosis can be emotionally challenging. The constant fear of falling and breaking a bone creates persistent anxiety, which can lead to chronic stress, further worsening the condition. Many patients feel overwhelmed by their diagnosis, experiencing a loss of control that can contribute to depression.

Osteoporosis also affects social interactions. Activities once enjoyed, like dancing or hiking, may now feel too risky, leading to social withdrawal and isolation. This avoidance of social activities can strain relationships with family and friends, and relying on others for support can sometimes lead to feelings of being a burden.

Managing these emotional challenges is essential. Stress relief techniques, such as deep breathing, mindfulness, and progressive muscle relaxation, can help reduce anxiety. Building a strong support network of family, friends, or members of a local support group can provide both emotional and practical help. Seeking professional counseling, particularly Cognitive Behavioral Therapy (CBT), can be especially effective in managing anxiety and depression linked to chronic illness.

Chapter 2: Diagnosis and Medical Testing

Imagine waking up with a sharp pain in your back, dismissing it as part

of aging or an awkward night's sleep. Weeks pass, and the pain persists. You notice your jeans don't fit like they used to, despite no weight gain. You've lost height. These subtle changes are how osteoporosis often begins—quietly and without fanfare.

Osteoporosis is often called the "silent disease" because early stages typically have no symptoms. One of the first signs is unexplained, persistent back pain, which may result from undetected micro-fractures in the spine. Over time, this can lead to a hunched posture and severe back issues.

Another early indicator is gradual height loss, caused by the weakening and compression of spinal vertebrae. You may notice that reaching for high shelves becomes more complicated or that your clothes seem longer. Additionally, fractures from low-impact activities—like slipping on a rug or bending over—are warning signs that your bones are becoming less dense.

Women, especially postmenopausal, are more prone to these symptoms due to hormonal changes, while men experience a slower decline in bone density. Men may not realize they have osteoporosis until a fracture occurs, often later in life, leading to delayed diagnosis and treatment. Detecting these signs early allows for timely intervention, helping preserve bone strength and prevent fractures.

Self-Assessment Tools

Self-assessment tools, including online risk calculators, can help you gauge your osteoporosis risk by asking about factors like age, gender, family history, and past fractures. While these tools can't replace professional advice, they can prompt a discussion with your doctor. Additionally, checklists can guide you in discussing symptoms with your healthcare provider, ensuring you address all critical aspects such as diet, physical activity, and recent physical changes.

Early diagnosis and proactive treatment can make a significant difference in managing osteoporosis, preventing further bone deterioration, and supporting a healthier, more active life.

Diagnostic Tools and Techniques

The most commonly used diagnostic tool for osteoporosis is the DEXA scan, which measures bone mineral density (BMD). It provides clear images of areas most prone to fractures, such as the spine, hip, and forearm, allowing doctors to assess bone health and determine the necessary treatment plan.

Another diagnostic tool is quantitative ultrasound, which uses sound waves to assess bone density, typically on the heel. It's more affordable and portable than the DEXA scan, making it convenient for preliminary assessments. However, it's not as accurate as DEXA, and if results indicate low bone density, your doctor will likely recommend a DEXA scan for a more precise evaluation.

CT scans (computed tomography) can also measure bone density but are less commonly used due to higher radiation exposure and cost. These scans provide detailed images of bone structure and density. They are typically reserved for cases where other tests are inconclusive or when more precise imaging is needed, such as for surgical planning.

Peripheral bone density tests assess bone density in peripheral areas of the body, such as the wrist, fingers, or heel. These tests are faster and cheaper than the central DEXA scans but are less detailed. They can be used for preliminary assessments or in cases where a full-body DEXA scan is not possible. However, they should not be used as the only method to determine the presence of osteoporosis.

Magnetic resonance imaging, commonly known as MRI, can give you images of bones without having to use radiation. Although MRI is not widely used to diagnose osteoporosis, it can help determine the quality of the bone and identify fractures that cannot be seen on X-rays or DEXA scans. It helps give a detailed view of the structure of bones, which can be quite beneficial in formulating treatment plans.

Diagnosis and Medical Testing

The DEXA scan is the gold standard for diagnosing osteoporosis due to its accuracy in evaluating bone mineral density (BMD) at critical sites like the spine and hip. While it involves low radiation levels, it offers the most precise assessment of bone health. In contrast, quantitative ultrasound is a quicker, more affordable option without radiation but is less accurate and primarily used for initial screening. CT scans and MRIs provide detailed bone images but come with higher costs and radiation exposure.

The type of diagnostic tool used depends on individual risk factors. A DEXA scan is usually recommended for its precision in high-risk individuals. Ultrasound and peripheral bone density tests may serve as screening tools, especially when DEXA scans are unavailable. CT scans or MRIs may be used in more complex cases requiring detailed imaging.

Understanding Bone Density Scans (DEXA)

A DEXA scan uses two X-ray beams to measure bone density. It focuses on areas prone to fractures, such as the hips and spine, and is a noninvasive, pain-free procedure. Results include T-scores and Z-scores, which help assess the risk of fractures and guide treatment. While there are concerns about radiation, the exposure from a DEXA scan is minimal—lower than that from a chest X-ray.

The T-score compares your bone density to that of a young, healthy individual, while the Z-score compares it to others of your age, sex, and height. A T-score of -1.0 or higher is normal, while a lower score indicates bone loss. Bone turnover markers, such as alkaline phosphatase and osteocalcin, can provide additional insights into bone metabolism, helping assess treatment effectiveness.

Case Studies

Jane - Rediscovering Strength Through Community Support

At 52, Jane was diagnosed with osteoporosis after experiencing a wrist fracture from a minor fall. The news was shocking; she had always led an active lifestyle and assumed her bones were strong. Jane's first reaction was fear—fear of more fractures, fear of losing her independence, and fear of what the diagnosis meant for her future. However, Jane refused to let her diagnosis define her.

Initially, Jane felt isolated, unsure of where to turn. She tried to continue her usual routines, but her increasing fear of falling left her less active and more withdrawn. After a few months, she knew she needed to act, so she reached out to a local osteoporosis support group. This decision changed her life.

Jane started attending weekly exercise classes designed for people with osteoporosis. The instructor introduced her to weight-bearing exercises and Tai Chi, which improved her balance, strength, and confidence. Additionally, Jane found a sense of community in the group. Sharing her fears and triumphs with others who truly understood her experience helped Jane regain control of her life.

Through her journey, Jane also focused on her diet, working with a nutritionist to incorporate more calcium-rich foods and ensure she was getting enough vitamin D. She took small steps—adjusting her daily routine to include healthier meals and finding ways to stay active within her limits.

Key Takeaways:

- Joining a support group and participating in osteoporosis-specific exercise programs can enhance both physical and emotional well-being.
- A strong support network, including professionals like nutritionists, can help develop a tailored health plan that complements medical treatment.
- Small, consistent lifestyle changes, such as adjusting your diet and engaging in safe physical activity, are crucial to managing osteoporosis

Michael - A Firefighter's Path to Recovery and Prevention

Michael, a 64-year-old retired firefighter, was no stranger to physical challenges. However, when a seemingly small slip on wet pavement resulted in a hip fracture, he was diagnosed with osteoporosis. Like many men, Michael had never considered that he might be at risk. The diagnosis felt like a heavy blow to his self-image as a strong, physically capable man.

After surgery to repair his hip, Michael's doctor recommended a bone density scan, which confirmed that he had osteoporosis. Initially frustrated and discouraged, Michael had to confront the fact that this condition would require significant lifestyle adjustments.

Determined to regain his strength, Michael began working with a physical therapist to create a structured exercise routine that included resistance training and balance exercises. He focused on low-impact activities like swimming and cycling, which helped him rebuild muscle without putting too much strain on his bones.

Michael also made important dietary changes. He increased his intake of calcium and magnesium-rich foods, such as leafy greens, nuts, and seeds, and began taking vitamin D supplements as his doctor advised. Additionally, he stopped smoking—a habit he'd struggled with for years—recognizing how it weakened his bones.

Michael's experience as a firefighter had taught him resilience, and he applied that same determination to his osteoporosis journey. Over time, he not only recovered from his fracture but also became a strong advocate for men's bone health, encouraging others to get screened and make bone health a priority.

Key Takeaways:

- Men are often unaware of their risk for osteoporosis, making regular bone density screenings necessary for early diagnosis.
- Recovery from a fracture requires both physical therapy and lifestyle changes, such as improving diet and quitting harmful habits like smoking.
- Strength and resilience come from physical capability and the determination to make long-term changes that support bone health.

Maria - Traditional Wisdom Meets Modern Medicine

At 70, Maria was diagnosed with osteoporosis after experiencing multiple minor fractures. Raised in a family that valued traditional remedies, she was initially hesitant to rely on medications. However, her fractures made it clear that she needed a plan that combined both her cultural heritage and modern treatment options.

Maria sought guidance from her healthcare provider but also consulted with an Ayurvedic practitioner, who introduced her to natural herbs like ashwagandha and turmeric to support her bone health. Maria integrated these into her routine, alongside her prescribed medication, and noticed improvements in her overall well-being.

In addition, Maria embraced yoga to improve her balance and flexibility. Although she had learned yoga in her youth, she had not practiced it regularly for years. As part of her osteoporosis management, she rediscovered the gentle poses that helped strengthen her muscles and joints without putting excessive pressure on her bones.

Her approach blended traditional remedies with medical guidance, proving that you don't have to choose one over the other. With her doctor monitoring her progress, Maria safely integrated her Ayurvedic supplements while adhering to her prescribed treatments.

Key Takeaways:

- Blending traditional remedies with modern medical treatments can offer a holistic approach to managing osteoporosis.
- Consulting with healthcare providers to ensure safety is critical when incorporating natural supplements alongside prescription medication.
- Gentle exercises like yoga can be highly beneficial for maintaining balance, flexibility, and overall bone health, especially for older adults.

Imani - Advocacy Through Adversity

Imani, a vibrant 37-year-old woman, was diagnosed with osteoporosis due to a rare genetic condition. The diagnosis came after a fracture from a fall during a simple jog—a wake-up call for Imani, who had always been physically active. Unlike most people with osteoporosis, Imani's youth made the diagnosis even more unexpected, and she struggled with the stigma of having a condition typically associated with older adults.

Imani initially felt angry and frustrated but quickly turned her emotions into advocacy. She created a blog to share her story and connect with others who, like her, faced the emotional and physical challenges of osteoporosis at a younger age. Her blog gained traction, and soon, she had a supportive online community that shared resources, tips, and stories of resilience.

With her doctor's support, Imani developed a comprehensive treatment plan that included bisphosphonates to strengthen her bones and strength training exercises to enhance her muscle mass. She also focused on maintaining a balanced calcium-rich diet, opting for plant-based sources due to her lactose intolerance.

Imani's advocacy work has empowered many others with osteoporosis to share their stories and actively manage their health. She thrives by balancing her treatment plan with her passion for raising awareness.

Key Takeaways:

- Younger individuals with osteoporosis may face unique emotional challenges, including stigma and isolation, but advocacy and community can provide support.
- Raising awareness and sharing personal experiences can empower others to take control of their health.
- A tailored treatment plan, including medication, exercise, and dietary modifications, can help younger individuals manage osteoporosis effectively.

Ayesha - Bridging Cultures to Find Balance

Ayesha, a 58-year-old woman of Middle Eastern descent, was diagnosed with osteoporosis after her doctor noticed signs of significant bone loss during a routine checkup. Having grown up in a family where traditional health remedies were commonly used, Ayesha felt conflicted about starting medication.

Her doctor recommended bisphosphonates to manage her condition, but Ayesha wanted to explore natural remedies first. She consulted her family, who suggested trying calcium-rich seeds like sesame and chia, staples in her cultural diet. Ayesha incorporated these into her meals and fortified plant-based milk as she struggled with lactose intolerance.

To address her concerns about mobility and balance, Ayesha took inspiration from Middle Eastern dance, also known as belly dancing. She found a local class and discovered that the gentle movements improved her core strength and flexibility, reducing her risk of falls. This cultural connection helped her physically and emotionally, reconnecting her to a part of her identity.

Ayesha's ability to combine modern treatments with cultural practices allowed her to find a balance that worked for her. She continues to thrive today, blending her traditional values with modern osteoporosis care.

Key Takeaways:

- Cultural traditions can offer valuable insights and tools for managing bone health, especially when combined with modern treatments.
- Movement-based activities, like dance, can improve balance and strength while providing emotional and cultural benefits.
- Exploring a mix of traditional and modern remedies can lead to a personalized, effective osteoporosis management plan.

John - Late Diagnosis and the Path to Recovery

At 67, John's active lifestyle was abruptly interrupted by a fall that resulted in a fractured vertebra. It wasn't until this incident that he was diagnosed with osteoporosis, a condition he had unknowingly lived with for years. For John, the late diagnosis felt like a setback, but he was determined to rebuild his health.

John worked closely with his healthcare provider to develop a comprehensive recovery plan. This included taking anabolic medications to stimulate bone growth and enrolling in a physical rehabilitation program to rebuild his strength and mobility. He also began incorporating Tai Chi into his routine to improve his balance and prevent future falls.

As part of his new lifestyle, John adopted a plant-based diet rich in calcium, magnesium, and vitamin D. He swapped out his usual fast-food meals for home-cooked dishes featuring leafy greens, beans, and fortified alternatives.

Over time, John's dedication to his treatment and lifestyle changes helped him recover his mobility and confidence. He now advocates for early osteoporosis screening, particularly for men, to ensure others don't face

Monitoring Bone Health

Regular monitoring is essential for managing osteoporosis, as it provides crucial insights into your bone health over time. The DEXA (Dual-Energy X-ray Absorptiometry) scan, considered the gold standard for measuring bone mineral density (BMD), is recommended every two years for postmenopausal women and men over 70. This simple, non-invasive scan helps assess the current state of your bones, providing valuable information on whether your bone density is improving, stabilizing, or declining. For individuals at higher risk, such as those with a history of fractures, specific medical conditions, or long-term steroid use, more frequent monitoring may be necessary. This allows for early detection of any adverse changes and timely adjustments to the treatment plan.

However, while the DEXA scan is vital, it's only one piece of the puzzle. Bone turnover markers, which are proteins or enzymes found in your blood or urine, offer additional insights into the rate at which your bones are breaking down and rebuilding. These markers help assess whether the treatment effectively slows bone loss or increases bone formation. For instance, C-telopeptide (CTX) and procollagen type 1 N-terminal propeptide (P1NP) are commonly measured markers that indicate the activity of bone turnover. Monitoring these markers provides an earlier indicator of how well your body is responding to therapy, often before changes in bone density are visible on a DEXA scan.

In addition to these tests, regular physical exams are an essential component of managing osteoporosis. Your healthcare provider will assess factors such as posture, mobility, balance, and overall strength. These assessments are particularly important for identifying changes that might increase the risk of falls and fractures. A physical exam can also help detect spinal deformities, such as kyphosis, which can result from vertebral fractures associated with osteoporosis.

Furthermore, your doctor may evaluate other health factors that contribute to bone health, such as hormone levels (particularly in postmenopausal women), calcium and vitamin D levels, and overall nutritional status. These routine assessments allow your healthcare team to take a holistic approach, ensuring that all contributing factors to bone health are addressed, whether through medication, supplements, lifestyle adjustments, or dietary changes.

Regular monitoring not only tracks progress but also empowers you to make informed decisions about your treatment. Whether it's deciding when to intensify therapy, exploring new treatment options, or making small adjustments to your routine, having a clear picture of your bone health enables proactive management of osteoporosis. Regular communication with your healthcare provider is key, as they will interpret these results in the context of your overall health, adjusting your treatment plan as needed to ensure the best outcomes.

By staying vigilant with DEXA scans, bone turnover markers, and physical exams, you're taking a proactive step in protecting your bone health and minimizing the risk of fractures, giving you greater control over your osteoporosis management.

Discussing Results with Your Doctor

When it comes to managing osteoporosis, conversation with your doctor about your test results is crucial. Preparing for your appointment can help you get the most out of this discussion. Start by noting down any specific questions you may have about your recent tests. For instance, understanding the difference between T-scores and Z-scores can be confusing but is essential for assessing your bone health. The T-score compares your bone density to that of a healthy young adult, while the Z-score compares it to people of your age, gender, and size. Knowing what these numbers mean in relation to your overall bone health will help you understand the severity of your condition and guide decisions about your treatment.

It's also important to share any new or worsening symptoms you've experienced, such as back pain or height loss, which can be indicative of vertebral fractures—a common yet sometimes silent consequence of osteoporosis. These symptoms provide important context that your doctor will consider when assessing your overall bone health. Even subtle changes in posture or unexplained pain should be discussed, as they could signal underlying issues that might not appear immediately on a DEXA scan.

Beyond the physical aspects, it's essential to address the emotional impact of living with osteoporosis openly. Many individuals find the diagnosis overwhelming, often feeling anxious about the possibility of fractures or changes in their independence. Let your doctor know if you're feeling anxious, fearful, or even depressed about managing your condition. They may be able to provide resources such as counseling or support groups that can help you manage the emotional toll of osteoporosis. Addressing these concerns also ensures that your treatment plan accounts for your mental and physical well-being.

When reviewing your results, be proactive in discussing the next steps for your treatment. Ask about potential treatment options, whether they involve medication, supplements, or more holistic approaches like physical therapy. Discuss the benefits and possible side effects of any prescribed medications, and don't hesitate to bring up any lifestyle changes you could make to complement your medical treatment. For example, you might ask about incorporating weight-bearing exercises or adjusting your diet to improve calcium and vitamin D intake. Collaborating with your doctor on these lifestyle changes ensures that your treatment plan is well-rounded and tailored to your individual needs.

If you're uncertain about any recommendations, don't be afraid to seek a second opinion. It's vital that you feel confident and comfortable with the course of treatment you're pursuing. A second opinion can provide reassurance or offer new insights that could enhance your care.

Lastly, if you feel that additional therapies—like physical therapy—could benefit your mobility, balance, or overall strength, suggest these options to your doctor. Physical therapy is often an invaluable resource in helping manage osteoporosis, particularly in preventing falls and improving muscle strength, both of which can reduce the risk of fractures. Your doctor can help coordinate these services and ensure they are covered as part of your treatment plan.

By preparing for your appointment, asking the right questions, and advocating for your health, you can have a productive conversation with your doctor and more effectively manage osteoporosis.

Chapter 3: Medical Treatments and Alternatives

I remember when my mom first experienced severe osteoporosis symptoms. It was a difficult time for our family. We spent hours discussing her treatment options, navigating a maze of medical information, and trying to make sense of terms that were new and overwhelming. The fear of what this condition could mean for her future was daunting, but we knew we had to face it head-on.

The process started with a series of appointments. Her doctor explained the various medical treatments available, from bisphosphonates and hormone therapies to newer options like biologics. Each came with its benefits and potential side effects, leaving us with decisions that felt as weighty as the diagnosis itself. For my mom, it wasn't simply a matter of swallowing a pill or taking an injection; she wanted to fully understand what each treatment meant for her overall health, not just her bones.

We quickly learned that managing osteoporosis went beyond the doctor's office. It wasn't just about choosing a medication; it was about understanding the condition in total—how her lifestyle might need to change, the long-term effects, and how she could stay active and independent despite the challenges. Dietary changes became a cornerstone of her plan. We researched foods rich in calcium, magnesium, and vitamin D, creating meals that felt less like a chore and more like an empowering step toward healing.

I hadn't fully anticipated the emotional toll of osteoporosis. I saw how my mom grappled with the fear of falling or the frustration of needing to adjust her daily routines. It wasn't just her bones that needed strengthening—her confidence did, too. We explored alternatives like yoga and tai chi, which not only improved her balance and strength but also became a source of relaxation and mindfulness.

It took time for her to come to terms with the diagnosis. I remember how we sat together, combing through materials on treatment plans and alternatives, wondering if there were natural remedies she could try or lifestyle adjustments that might help lessen the impact of osteoporosis. Herbal remedies like red clover and black cohosh surfaced in our research, though we knew they needed to be approached cautiously. We also found studies on the potential of supplements like collagen and probiotics to support bone health, which became a point of hope in our journey.

This experience reminded me that managing osteoporosis is deeply personal. It's not just about picking the proper medication—it's about addressing the emotional, mental, and physical adjustments that come with such a diagnosis. Every decision felt like a puzzle piece, slowly coming together to create a picture of resilience and adaptability. My mom's journey showed me that the path to managing osteoporosis isn't one-size-fits-all—it's as unique as the individuals it affects.

Overview of Osteoporosis Medications

Osteoporosis treatments fall into several main categories: bisphosphonates, selective estrogen receptor modulators (SERMs), calcitonin, and parathyroid hormone analogs. Each works differently to improve bone mass.

1. **Bisphosphonates** are the most commonly prescribed medications. They slow down bone resorption (bone breakdown), helping maintain or improve bone density. Common bisphosphonates include alendronate (Fosamax), risedronate (Actonel), and ibandronate (Boniva), which are available in tablet form or as injections.

2. **Selective Estrogen Receptor Modulators (SERMs)**, such as Raloxifene (Evista), act like estrogen in bones without affecting other tissues. SERMs reduce bone resorption, particularly useful for postmenopausal women who cannot take hormone replacement therapy (HRT).

3. **Calcitonin** is a hormone that regulates calcium levels and prevents bone resorption. Synthetic calcitonin (like Miacalcin and Fortical) is available as a nasal spray or injection, making it easy to use when other treatments aren't suitable.

4. **Parathyroid hormone analogs**, such as Teriparatide (Forteo) and Abaloparatide (Tymlos), are unique because they stimulate bone formation. These daily injections are especially effective for patients with severe osteoporosis or multiple fractures.

Types of Osteoporosis Medications

Medication Type	Common Brands	Mechanism of Action	Administration
Bisphosphonates	Fosamax, Actonel, Boniva	Slows bone resorption	Oral tablets or injections
SERMs	Evista	Acts like estrogen in bones, reduces bone loss	Oral tablets
Calcitonin	Miacalcin, Fortical	Inhibits bone resorption	Nasal spray or injection
Parathyroid hormone analogs	Forteo, Tymlos	Stimulates new bone formation	Daily injections

Understanding how each medication works will help you and your healthcare provider make informed decisions about managing osteoporosis.

Choosing the right osteoporosis medication depends on factors like overall health, osteoporosis severity, and personal preferences. Options range from daily tablets to monthly injections or nasal sprays, all aimed at improving bone density and preventing fractures, allowing you to stay active.

Osteoporosis medications, such as Fosamax (a bisphosphonate), have been shown to reduce vertebral fractures by 50% and hip fractures by nearly 40%. These medications can significantly improve bone density, especially during the first year of treatment.

However, side effects are a consideration. Common issues include gastrointestinal discomfort, such as nausea or heartburn. Rare but serious risks include atypical femoral fractures (spontaneous thigh bone fractures) and osteonecrosis of the jaw (bone death in the jaw, often related to dental procedures). Regular monitoring through bone density tests (like DEXA scans) and blood tests for calcium levels is essential to track treatment effectiveness and prevent complications.

Extended use of medications, like bisphosphonates, often involves a "drug holiday" after five years to minimize risks, though high-risk patients may need more prolonged treatment. A drug holiday requires careful supervision, with routine check-ups to ensure bone health remains stable.

Anabolic Therapies for Bone Building

Anabolic therapies like Teriparatide (Forteo) and Abaloparatide (Tymlos) are administered through easy-to-use daily injections, usually for up to two years. These treatments stimulate bone formation by activating osteoblasts (cells that form new bone), significantly increasing bone mineral density, especially in the hip and spine. The improvements lead to fewer fractures and a better quality of life. However, there are some long-term safety concerns, such as the rare risk of osteosarcoma (bone cancer), though this hasn't been reported in humans at the recommended dosage.

While anabolic therapies are highly effective, they are expensive, and not all insurance plans fully cover the cost. Since the treatment lasts only two years, patients must switch to antiresorptive drugs afterward to maintain the new bone density gains.

Natural Supplements: Calcium and Vitamin D

Calcium is vital for bone health, as 99% of it is stored in bones. The recommended daily intake for adults is 1,000–1,200 mg. Vitamin D enhances calcium absorption, with a daily recommendation of 600–800 IU for adults. Sources include sunlight, fortified foods, and supplements.

Calcium supplements come in two forms: calcium carbonate, which requires food for absorption, and calcium citrate, which is easier to absorb and can be taken on an empty stomach. Vitamin D3 is more effective than D2 in raising vitamin D levels. When taking supplements, be mindful not to take them with iron-rich foods or medications that may interfere with absorption.

Despite myths, moderate calcium supplementation does not typically cause kidney stones. Drinking enough water and avoiding excess salt helps reduce risks. Always consult your doctor to avoid interactions between supplements and medications.

Balancing Medication with Natural Remedies

Combining medication with natural remedies can effectively manage osteoporosis, enhancing the benefits of both treatments while promoting a holistic approach to bone health. Medications like bisphosphonates are designed to slow bone loss and increase bone density, providing a critical foundation for osteoporosis management. However, their effectiveness can be significantly enhanced when paired with a calcium-rich diet and adequate vitamin D intake. Calcium and vitamin D work synergistically to support bone structure, and they are readily available in dietary sources like leafy greens, dairy products, fortified foods, or supplements when needed. Together, these nutrients help maximize the medication's ability to rebuild and fortify bones.

Similarly, selective estrogen receptor modulators (SERMs) are most effective when combined with regular physical activity. Weight-bearing exercises such as walking, hiking, or resistance training stimulate bone formation while improving balance and muscle strength. Low-impact activities like yoga and Tai Chi also enhance coordination, reduce the risk of falls, and provide added mental health benefits.

An individualized treatment plan is essential to achieving the best results when balancing pharmacotherapy with natural remedies. Regular consultations with healthcare providers ensure that medications, dietary adjustments, and lifestyle changes are tailored to your specific needs. This holistic approach allows both interventions to work harmoniously, optimizing bone health while fostering a sustainable and active lifestyle.

By integrating medication with natural strategies, individuals with osteoporosis can manage the condition effectively and improve overall quality of life. This dual approach emphasizes the importance of treating the body as a whole, supporting long-term health and independence.

Exploring Global Natural Remedies

Traditional practices and natural remedies have been developed around the world to support bone health and complement conventional osteoporosis treatments. These approaches, often rooted in centuries of cultural wisdom, provide unique insights into maintaining strong bones and preventing fractures.

- Traditional Chinese Medicine (TCM): TCM emphasizes holistic balance and often incorporates herbs like ginseng and Rehmannia to strengthen bones and improve overall vitality. Additionally, practices such as Tai Chi combine physical movement with mindfulness to enhance balance, improve muscle strength, and reduce the risk of falls—key benefits for individuals with osteoporosis. Research supports Tai Chi's effectiveness in enhancing stability and preventing fractures, making it a valuable addition to any treatment plan.

- Ayurveda: This ancient Indian practice focuses on harmonizing the body's energies. Herbs such as turmeric, known for its anti-inflammatory properties, and ashwagandha, which supports bone density, are often used in Ayurvedic remedies. Ayurveda also promotes yoga for flexibility, strength, and balance, offering a low-impact way to improve mobility while nurturing the mind-body connection.

- European Herbal Remedies: In Europe, plants like nettles, horsetail, and red clover are traditionally used for their bone-supporting properties. Nettles are rich in calcium and magnesium, while horsetail contains silica, a mineral that helps strengthen the bone matrix. Coupled with the Mediterranean diet—renowned for its emphasis on vegetables, fruits, whole grains, and healthy fats—these remedies offer a nutrient-rich approach to sustaining bone health.

Incorporating these global remedies into your osteoporosis management plan can complement conventional treatments and promote overall well-being. For instance, studies have shown that ginseng may increase bone density, while Tai Chi improves balance and enhances mental clarity, fostering a holistic sense of health.

Before starting any new supplements or practices, always consult your healthcare provider. Quality control is crucial, as not all products meet rigorous safety standards. Begin with low dosages and gradually adjust to suit your needs, ensuring these remedies harmonize with your existing treatments. When approached thoughtfully, global natural remedies can enhance your journey to stronger bones and better health.

Chapter 4: Nutrition for Bone Health

Imagine sitting alone at the dining table, flipping through a photo album. You see your mom, vibrant and full of life, but then remember how osteoporosis later made everyday activities difficult for her. It's in these quiet moments that the connection between diet and bone health becomes undeniable—what we eat directly impacts the strength and resilience of our bones.

Think of bones as living structures that are constantly breaking down and being rebuilt. Like constructing a sturdy house, they need the right materials to remain strong over time. Calcium is the cornerstone, providing the bulk of bone strength, while Vitamin D acts as the foreman, ensuring calcium is absorbed effectively. Beyond these essentials, magnesium and phosphorus play supporting roles, reinforcing the bone matrix. Vitamin K helps to form and maintain bone tissue, while protein serves as the scaffolding that holds everything together. Without these critical nutrients, bones can become brittle, increasing the risk of fractures and making recovery slower and more complicated.

The challenge isn't just knowing what to eat—it's creating a sustainable way to incorporate these nutrients into everyday life. For example, leafy greens like kale, collard greens, and spinach are excellent sources of calcium and magnesium. Fortified plant-based milk or dairy products can fill in any gaps, especially for those who are lactose intolerant or prefer non-dairy options. Fatty fish such as salmon and mackerel provide Vitamin D and omega-3 fatty acids, which support overall bone and joint health. Even tiny seeds like chia and sesame punch above their weight, offering both calcium and magnesium in compact, versatile forms.

Diets like the Mediterranean diet, rich in vegetables, fruits, whole grains, and healthy fats, have emerged as champions for bone health. This way of eating provides a wealth of vitamins and minerals while reducing the intake of bone-depleting substances. In contrast, high sodium levels, often found in processed and fast foods, can leach calcium from the bones, weakening them over time. Caffeine, when consumed in excess, may also contribute to calcium loss, although moderate intake in the context of a well-balanced diet is less concerning.

Hydration, often overlooked, also plays a role in bone health. Staying hydrated supports overall cellular function, including the repair and maintenance of bone tissue. Adding bone-friendly ingredients like a splash of citrus juice to your water can provide Vitamin C, which aids in collagen production—a key component of bone structure.

Reducing processed foods and opting for whole, nutrient-dense options can significantly improve bone strength. Simple substitutions, like replacing refined grains with quinoa or farro, swapping sugary snacks for nuts and dried fruits, or using olive oil instead of butter, can make a tangible difference. Even fermented foods like yogurt and kimchi, rich in probiotics, support gut health, which is increasingly linked to better nutrient absorption and bone density.

Ultimately, the goal isn't just about meeting daily nutrient requirements—it's about creating a dietary pattern that supports your bones throughout your life. Each meal is an opportunity to strengthen your body and prevent the silent progression of osteoporosis. By making informed choices, you can lay the foundation for a future where mobility, strength, and independence remain within your grasp.

Calcium-Rich Foods and How to Include them in your Diet

Dairy products are excellent sources of calcium:

- 1 cup of milk = 300 mg calcium
- 8 oz yogurt = 400 mg calcium
- 1 oz cheddar cheese = 200 mg calcium

Non-dairy options include:

- 1 cup cooked kale = 177 mg calcium
- 1 oz almonds = 75 mg calcium
- 1 tbsp sesame seeds = 88 mg calcium
- 3 oz sardines = 325 mg calcium

Incorporating calcium-rich foods into meals is easy. Add spinach or kale to smoothies, enjoy almond snacks, or use tofu in stir-fries. Here are some recipes for you to try:

Calcium-Rich Smoothie Bowl

This vibrant smoothie bowl is packed with calcium and other essential nutrients for bone health.

Ingredients:

- 1 cup fortified almond milk (450 mg calcium)
- 1/2 cup plain Greek yogurt (100 mg calcium)
- 1/2 cup frozen kale or spinach (30 mg calcium)
- 1/2 banana
- 1/2 cup frozen mixed berries
- 1 tbsp chia seeds (60 mg calcium)
- 1 tbsp almond butter (40 mg calcium)
- 1 tbsp granola (optional for texture)

Instructions:

1. Blend the almond milk, Greek yogurt, kale or spinach, banana, and berries until smooth.
2. Pour into a bowl and top with chia seeds, almond butter, and granola.
3. Serve immediately and enjoy this calcium-rich, energizing start to your day!

Baked Salmon with Sesame Kale

This recipe combines the calcium benefits of leafy greens with the vitamin D from salmon, providing a nutrient-packed meal for bone health.

Ingredients:

- 2 salmon fillets (570 IU vitamin D per serving)
- 4 cups kale, chopped (177 mg calcium per cup)
- 1 tbsp sesame seeds (88 mg calcium)
- 1 tbsp olive oil
- 1 clove garlic, minced
- 1 tbsp lemon juice
- Salt and pepper to taste

Instructions:

1. Preheat the oven to 375°F (190°C). Season the salmon fillets with salt, pepper, and a drizzle of olive oil.

2. Bake the salmon for 15-20 minutes or until it flakes easily with a fork.

3. Meanwhile, sauté the garlic in olive oil over medium heat. Add the chopped kale and cook until wilted, about 3-5 minutes.

4. Sprinkle sesame seeds over the kale and season with lemon juice, salt, and pepper.

5. Serve the baked salmon on a bed of sesame kale.

Chickpea, Spinach, and Quinoa Stir-Fry

This dish is loaded with plant-based calcium and magnesium, ideal for vegans or anyone looking for a nutrient-dense meal.

Ingredients:

- 1 cup cooked quinoa (31 mg calcium)
- 1 can chickpeas, drained and rinsed (210 mg calcium)
- 3 cups spinach, chopped (245 mg calcium)
- 1/2 red bell pepper, sliced
- 1 tbsp olive oil
- 2 garlic cloves, minced
- 1 tsp cumin
- 1/2 tsp paprika
- Salt and pepper to taste

Instructions:

1. Heat the olive oil in a pan over medium heat. Add garlic and sauté until fragrant.
2. Add the bell pepper and cook for 2-3 minutes.
3. Stir in the chickpeas, spinach, cumin, paprika, salt, and pepper. Cook until the spinach is wilted.
4. Mix in the cooked quinoa and stir well to combine.
5. Serve warm, garnished with a sprinkle of fresh herbs, if desired.

Tofu and Broccoli Stir-Fry with Almonds

Tofu, broccoli, and almonds boost calcium in this flavorful and easy-to-make stir-fry.

Ingredients:

- 1/2 block firm tofu, cubed (430 mg calcium)
- 2 cups broccoli florets (86 mg calcium)
- 1/4 cup sliced almonds (75 mg calcium)
- 1 tbsp sesame oil
- 2 tbsp soy sauce (low sodium)
- 1 tsp grated ginger
- 1 garlic clove, minced
- 1 tbsp sesame seeds (optional)
- Cooked brown rice for serving

Instructions:

1. Heat sesame oil in a large pan or wok over medium heat. Add the tofu and cook until golden brown on all sides. Remove and set aside.
2. In the same pan, sauté garlic and ginger for 1 minute.
3. Add the broccoli florets and stir-fry for 5 minutes, until tender but still crisp.
4. Return the tofu to the pan, add soy sauce, and stir to combine.
5. Sprinkle with sliced almonds and sesame seeds (optional) for added crunch and calcium.
6. Serve over brown rice.

Sardine and Avocado Toast

This quick and tasty meal provides a great source of calcium and vitamin D from the sardines and healthy fats from the avocado.

Ingredients:

- 1 can sardines (325 mg calcium)
- 1 ripe avocado
- 2 slices whole grain bread
- 1 tbsp lemon juice
- Salt and pepper to taste
- Red pepper flakes (optional)

Instructions:

1. Toast the bread slices to your liking.
2. Mash the avocado in a bowl, mixing in the lemon juice, salt, and pepper.
3. Spread the avocado mixture on the toast and top with sardines.
4. Sprinkle with red pepper flakes for a spicy kick, if desired.

Almond Butter and Banana Chia Pudding

A calcium-rich dessert that's easy to make and full of bone-boosting nutrients.

Ingredients:

- 1/2 cup chia seeds (300 mg calcium)
- 2 cups almond milk (900 mg calcium)
- 1 tbsp almond butter (40 mg calcium)
- 1 banana, sliced
- 1 tsp vanilla extract
- 1 tsp maple syrup (optional)

Instructions:

1. In a bowl, whisk together chia seeds, almond milk, almond butter, vanilla extract, and maple syrup (if using).
2. Let the mixture sit for 10 minutes, then whisk again to prevent clumping.
3. Cover and refrigerate for at least 4 hours or overnight.
4. Serve topped with banana slices.

These healthy recipes are packed with bone-supporting nutrients like calcium, vitamin D, magnesium, and protein. They're easy to prepare and delicious, making it simple to support bone health through everyday meals.

The Importance of Vitamin D

Vitamin D is essential for absorbing calcium, and its best source is sunlight. Fifteen to twenty minutes of sun exposure a few times a week can provide sufficient vitamin D. Food sources include fatty fish, like salmon, eggs, and fortified foods. However, supplements may be necessary for those living in regions with limited sun exposure.

Sample Meal Plans for Stronger Bones

- **Breakfast**: Fortified cereal with berries and milk (300 mg calcium, 100 IU vitamin D).

- **Lunch**: Salmon salad with greens and almonds (250 mg calcium, 400 IU vitamin D).

- **Dinner**: Kale and almond pesto pasta (350 mg calcium).

Spinach and Feta Stuffed Chicken Breast

This flavorful dish combines lean protein with calcium-rich spinach and feta, making it a perfect dinner for bone health.

Ingredients:

- 2 boneless, skinless chicken breasts
- 1 cup fresh spinach, chopped (60 mg calcium)
- 1/4 cup crumbled feta cheese (100 mg calcium)
- 1 tbsp olive oil
- 1 clove garlic, minced
- Salt and pepper to taste

Instructions:

1. Preheat the oven to 375°F (190°C).
2. Butterfly the chicken breasts by slicing them horizontally without cutting all the way through.
3. Heat olive oil in a pan and sauté garlic until fragrant. Add spinach and cook until wilted.
4. Mix the cooked spinach with feta cheese and stuff the mixture into the chicken breasts. Secure with toothpicks.
5. Place the chicken in a baking dish, season with salt and pepper, and bake for 20-25 minutes or until fully cooked.

Greek Yogurt Parfait with Almonds and Berries

This easy-to-make parfait is rich in calcium, protein, and antioxidants, perfect for breakfast or a snack.

Ingredients:

- 1 cup Greek yogurt (200 mg calcium)
- 1/4 cup granola
- 1/2 cup mixed berries (blueberries, strawberries, raspberries)
- 1 tbsp sliced almonds (75 mg calcium)
- 1 tsp honey (optional)

Instructions:

1. layer Greek yogurt, granola, and berries in a glass or bowl.
2. Top with sliced almonds and drizzle with honey, if desired.
3. Serve immediately for a refreshing and nutritious treat.

Roasted Brussels Sprouts with Tahini Drizzle

This simple side dish packs a calcium punch with the combination of Brussels sprouts and tahini.

Ingredients:

- 2 cups Brussels sprouts, halved (110 mg calcium)
- 1 tbsp olive oil
- Salt and pepper to taste
- 2 tbsp tahini (130 mg calcium)
- 1 tbsp lemon juice
- 1 clove garlic, minced
- 2 tbsp water

Instructions:

1. Preheat the oven to 400°F (200°C). Toss Brussels sprouts with olive oil, salt, and pepper, then spread them on a baking sheet.
2. Roast for 20-25 minutes, until golden and crispy.
3. In a small bowl, whisk together tahini, lemon juice, garlic, and water to make a smooth drizzle.
4. Serve the roasted Brussels sprouts with the tahini drizzle on top.

Calcium-Packed Veggie Pizza

This homemade pizza is a fun and delicious way to sneak in calcium with nutrient-dense toppings.

Ingredients:

- 1 whole-grain pizza crust
- 1/4 cup tomato sauce
- 1/2 cup shredded mozzarella cheese (180 mg calcium)
- 1/2 cup cooked broccoli florets (43 mg calcium)
- 1/4 cup sliced bell peppers
- 2 tbsp grated Parmesan cheese (55 mg calcium)
- 1 tsp Italian seasoning

Instructions:

1. Preheat the oven according to the pizza crust package instructions.
2. Spread tomato sauce evenly over the crust.
3. Sprinkle mozzarella cheese over the sauce, then add broccoli and bell peppers.
4. Top with Parmesan cheese and Italian seasoning.
5. Bake as directed, until the crust is golden and the cheese is bubbly.

Tofu Scramble with Kale and Mushrooms

This vegan-friendly scramble is packed with calcium, magnesium, and protein to support bone health.

Ingredients:

- 1/2 block firm tofu, crumbled (430 mg calcium)
- 2 cups kale, chopped (177 mg calcium)
- 1/2 cup mushrooms, sliced
- 1 tbsp olive oil
- 1/4 tsp turmeric
- 1/4 tsp paprika
- Salt and pepper to taste

Instructions:

1. Heat olive oil in a skillet over medium heat. Add mushrooms and cook until softened.
2. Stir in kale and cook until wilted.
3. Add crumbled tofu, turmeric, paprika, salt, and pepper. Cook for 5-7 minutes, stirring frequently.
4. Serve hot, paired with whole-grain toast or avocado slices, for a hearty, nutrient-packed breakfast or lunch.

Sweet Potato and Black Bean Tacos

These flavorful tacos provide plant-based calcium and vitamin C for better calcium absorption.

Ingredients:

- 1 medium sweet potato, diced (40 mg calcium)
- 1 cup canned black beans, drained and rinsed (50 mg calcium)
- 2 cups chopped spinach (122 mg calcium)
- 1 tbsp olive oil
- 1 tsp cumin
- 1/2 tsp chili powder
- 4 small corn tortillas
- 2 tbsp plain Greek yogurt (50 mg calcium)
- Lime wedges for serving

Instructions:

1. Preheat the oven to 400°F (200°C). Toss diced sweet potato with olive oil, cumin, and chili powder. Roast for 20 minutes or until tender.
2. Heat black beans in a pan over low heat.
3. Warm tortillas and layer with roasted sweet potato, spinach, and black beans.
4. Drizzle with Greek yogurt and serve with lime wedges.

Sardine Pasta with Lemon and Capers

This simple pasta dish offers a boost of calcium and vitamin D from sardines.

Ingredients:

- 1 can sardines, drained (325 mg calcium)
- 8 oz whole-grain spaghetti
- 1 tbsp olive oil
- 2 garlic cloves, minced
- 1 tbsp capers
- 1 tbsp lemon juice
- 1/4 cup Parmesan cheese, grated (110 mg calcium)
- Salt and pepper to taste

Instructions:

1. Cook spaghetti according to package instructions. Drain and set aside.
2. Heat olive oil in a skillet over medium heat. Sauté garlic until fragrant.
3. Add sardines, breaking them into pieces with a fork. Stir in capers and lemon juice.
4. Toss the cooked spaghetti in the skillet and mix well. Top with Parmesan cheese before serving.

Cottage Cheese and Berry Bowl

A quick and refreshing snack loaded with calcium and antioxidants.

Ingredients:

- 1 cup cottage cheese (200 mg calcium)
- 1/2 cup mixed berries (blueberries, strawberries, raspberries)
- 1 tbsp chia seeds (60 mg calcium)
- 1 tsp honey

Instructions:

1. In a bowl, layer cottage cheese and mixed berries.
2. Sprinkle with chia seeds and drizzle with honey.
3. Enjoy as a snack or light breakfast.

Broccoli and Cheddar Soup

This creamy soup is rich in calcium and vitamin K, essential for bone health.

Ingredients:

- 2 cups broccoli florets (86 mg calcium per cup)
- 1/2 cup shredded cheddar cheese (200 mg calcium)
- 2 cups low-sodium vegetable broth
- 1 cup milk (300 mg calcium)
- 1 tbsp olive oil
- 1/2 onion, diced
- 1 clove garlic, minced
- Salt and pepper to taste

Instructions:

1. Heat olive oil in a pot over medium heat. Sauté onion and garlic until softened.
2. Add broccoli and vegetable broth. Simmer until broccoli is tender, about 10 minutes.
3. Blend the soup until smooth using an immersion blender. Stir in milk and cheddar cheese until melted.
4. Season with salt and pepper before serving.

Kale and White Bean Salad

A quick and nutritious salad that combines calcium-rich kale with protein-packed beans.

Ingredients:

- 3 cups kale, chopped (177 mg calcium per cup)
- 1 cup canned white beans, drained and rinsed (100 mg calcium)
- 1/4 cup crumbled feta cheese (100 mg calcium)
- 1 tbsp olive oil
- 1 tbsp lemon juice
- Salt and pepper to taste

Instructions:

1. In a large bowl, massage kale with olive oil and lemon juice until tender.
2. Add white beans and feta cheese. Toss to combine.
3. Season with salt and pepper before serving.

Almond and Fig Overnight Oats

This make-ahead breakfast is a delicious way to start the day with calcium and fiber.

Ingredients:

- 1/2 cup rolled oats
- 1 cup almond milk (450 mg calcium)
- 1 tbsp almond butter (40 mg calcium)
- 2 dried figs, chopped (25 mg calcium)
- 1 tsp vanilla extract

Instructions:

1. In a jar or bowl, combine oats, almond milk, almond butter, figs, and vanilla extract.
2. Stir well, cover, and refrigerate overnight.
3. Serve cold or warm the next morning.

Spinach and Ricotta Stuffed Shells

A satisfying meal rich in calcium and iron from spinach and ricotta.

Ingredients:

- 12 jumbo pasta shells
- 2 cups fresh spinach, chopped (122 mg calcium per cup)
- 1 cup ricotta cheese (240 mg calcium)
- 1/2 cup marinara sauce
- 1/4 cup shredded mozzarella cheese (180 mg calcium)
- 1/4 tsp nutmeg
- Salt and pepper to taste

Instructions:

1. Preheat the oven to 375°F (190°C). Cook pasta shells according to package instructions. Drain and set aside.
2. In a bowl, mix spinach, ricotta cheese, nutmeg, salt, and pepper.
3. Stuff each pasta shell with the spinach-ricotta mixture. Place in a baking dish and top with marinara sauce and mozzarella cheese.
4. Bake for 20-25 minutes until bubbly and golden.

Lentil and Sweet Potato Stew

A hearty, calcium-packed stew full of plant-based nutrients.

Ingredients:

- 1 cup red lentils (40 mg calcium)
- 1 medium sweet potato, diced (40 mg calcium)
- 1 cup canned diced tomatoes
- 2 cups low-sodium vegetable broth
- 2 cups kale, chopped (177 mg calcium per cup)
- 1 tbsp olive oil
- 1 tsp turmeric
- 1 tsp cumin
- 1 clove garlic, minced
- Salt and pepper to taste

Instructions:

1. Heat olive oil in a pot over medium heat. Sauté garlic until fragrant.
2. Add sweet potatoes, turmeric, and cumin. Cook for 2–3 minutes.
3. Stir in lentils, tomatoes, and vegetable broth. Simmer for 20 minutes.
4. Add kale and cook until wilted. Season with salt and pepper before serving.

Cabbage and Carrot Slaw with Tahini Dressing

A refreshing slaw that's rich in calcium and vitamins.

Ingredients:

- 2 cups shredded cabbage (40 mg calcium)
- 1 cup shredded carrots
- 2 tbsp tahini (130 mg calcium)
- 1 tbsp lemon juice
- 1 tbsp olive oil
- 1 tsp honey
- Salt and pepper to taste

Instructions:

1. In a large bowl, combine shredded cabbage and carrots.
2. Whisk tahini, lemon juice, olive oil, honey, salt, and pepper in a small bowl.
3. Pour the dressing over the slaw and toss to combine. Serve as a side dish.

Baked Eggplant Parmesan

This calcium-rich dish uses baked eggplant as a healthy base.

Ingredients:

- 1 medium eggplant, sliced (20 mg calcium per cup)
- 1/2 cup marinara sauce
- 1/2 cup shredded mozzarella (180 mg calcium)
- 1/4 cup grated Parmesan cheese (55 mg calcium)
- 1/4 cup breadcrumbs
- 1 tsp Italian seasoning

Instructions:

1. Preheat oven to 375°F (190°C). Arrange eggplant slices on a baking sheet.
2. Top each slice with marinara sauce, mozzarella, Parmesan, breadcrumbs, and Italian seasoning.
3. Bake for 20–25 minutes until cheese is bubbly.

Sesame-Crusted Tofu Nuggets

A crunchy snack packed with plant-based calcium.

Ingredients:

- 1/2 block firm tofu, cubed (430 mg calcium)
- 1/4 cup sesame seeds (352 mg calcium)
- 2 tbsp soy sauce (low sodium)
- 1 tbsp olive oil
- 1/4 tsp garlic powder

Instructions:

1. Preheat oven to 400°F (200°C). Toss tofu cubes with soy sauce and garlic powder.
2. Coat each cube in sesame seeds. Arrange on a baking sheet and drizzle with olive oil.
3. Bake for 15–20 minutes, turning halfway through, until golden.

Baked Oatmeal with Almonds and Berries

A warm, calcium-rich breakfast that's easy to prepare in advance.

Ingredients:

- 2 cups rolled oats (120 mg calcium)
- 2 cups almond milk (450 mg calcium)
- 1/2 cup sliced almonds (150 mg calcium)
- 1 cup mixed berries
- 1 tsp vanilla extract
- 1 tsp cinnamon

Instructions:

1. Preheat oven to 375°F (190°C). Combine all ingredients in a large mixing bowl.
2. Pour the mixture into a greased baking dish.
3. Bake for 25–30 minutes until set. Serve warm or cold.

Swiss Chard and Mushroom Frittata

A nutrient-dense dish packed with calcium and vitamin D.

Ingredients:

- 4 eggs
- 1/2 cup Swiss chard, chopped (50 mg calcium)
- 1/2 cup sliced mushrooms
- 1/4 cup shredded cheddar (100 mg calcium)
- 1 tbsp olive oil
- Salt and pepper to taste

Instructions:

1. Preheat oven to 350°F (175°C). Heat olive oil in an oven-safe skillet over medium heat.
2. Sauté mushrooms and Swiss chard until softened.
3. Beat eggs, mix with cheddar, and pour into the skillet.
4. Bake for 15 minutes or until the frittata is set.

Orange and Almond Salad

A light and refreshing salad with a calcium boost from almonds.

Ingredients:

- 1 large orange, segmented
- 4 cups mixed greens (40 mg calcium)
- 1/4 cup sliced almonds (75 mg calcium)
- 2 tbsp olive oil
- 1 tbsp balsamic vinegar
- Salt and pepper to taste

Instructions:

1. In a large bowl, combine orange segments, mixed greens, and almonds.
2. Drizzle with olive oil and balsamic vinegar. Toss gently and serve.

Spaghetti Squash with Creamy Tahini Sauce

A low-carb dish packed with calcium and healthy fats.

Ingredients:

- 1 medium spaghetti squash
- 2 tbsp tahini (130 mg calcium)
- 1 tbsp lemon juice
- 1 clove garlic, minced
- 1/4 cup water
- 1/4 tsp paprika
- Salt and pepper to taste

Instructions:

1. Preheat oven to 400°F (200°C). Cut the squash in half and roast for 40 minutes.
2. In a small bowl, whisk tahini, lemon juice, garlic, water, paprika, salt, and pepper.
3. Scrape squash strands with a fork and toss with the tahini sauce.

Creamy Polenta with Roasted Vegetables

A comforting dish full of calcium and flavor.

Ingredients:

- 1 cup polenta (30 mg calcium)
- 2 cups milk (600 mg calcium)
- 1/2 cup Parmesan cheese (110 mg calcium)
- 1 cup roasted vegetables (zucchini, bell peppers, or broccoli)
- 1 tbsp olive oil
- Salt and pepper to taste

Instructions:

1. Heat milk in a saucepan and slowly whisk in polenta. Cook until creamy, about 10 minutes.
2. Stir in Parmesan cheese and season with salt and pepper.
3. Top with roasted vegetables and serve warm.

Indian-Style Spinach and Paneer Curry (Saag Paneer)

A classic Indian dish packed with calcium from spinach and paneer (Indian cottage cheese).

Ingredients:

- 2 cups fresh spinach, chopped (245 mg calcium)
- 1 cup paneer cubes (150 mg calcium)
- 1 medium onion, finely chopped
- 2 garlic cloves, minced
- 1 tsp grated ginger
- 1/2 tsp turmeric
- 1/2 tsp cumin seeds
- 1/2 cup plain Greek yogurt (100 mg calcium)
- 1 tbsp olive oil
- Salt to taste

Instructions:

1. Heat olive oil in a pan and sauté cumin seeds until aromatic. Add onion, garlic, and ginger; cook until golden.

2. Stir in turmeric and spinach. Cook until wilted, then blend into a smooth paste (optional).

3. Add paneer cubes and Greek yogurt, and simmer for 5 minutes. Season with salt before serving with rice or naan.

Mediterranean Chickpea and Tahini Salad

This Middle Eastern-inspired salad combines chickpeas and tahini for a creamy, calcium-rich dish.

Ingredients:

- 1 can chickpeas, drained and rinsed (210 mg calcium)
- 1/4 cup tahini (260 mg calcium)
- 1 tbsp lemon juice
- 1 clove garlic, minced
- 2 cups mixed greens (40 mg calcium)
- 1/2 cup cherry tomatoes, halved
- 1 tbsp olive oil
- Salt and pepper to taste

Instructions:

1. Whisk tahini, lemon juice, garlic, and olive oil in a small bowl to make the dressing.
2. Toss chickpeas, mixed greens, and cherry tomatoes in a large bowl.
3. Drizzle with the tahini dressing and season with salt and pepper before serving.

Japanese Miso Soup with Tofu and Wakame

A simple Japanese soup rich in calcium from tofu and seaweed.

Ingredients:

- 4 cups water
- 2 tbsp miso paste
- 1/2 block firm tofu, cubed (430 mg calcium)
- 1/4 cup dried wakame seaweed (40 mg calcium)
- 2 green onions, sliced

Instructions:

1. Bring water to a boil and stir in miso paste until dissolved.
2. Add tofu and wakame, and simmer for 5 minutes.
3. Garnish with green onions before serving.

Mexican Black Bean and Avocado Tostadas

A crispy and flavorful Mexican dish with plant-based calcium.

Ingredients:

- 4 small corn tortillas
- 1 cup black beans, mashed (50 mg calcium)
- 1 avocado, sliced
- 1/4 cup shredded cheddar cheese (100 mg calcium)
- 1/2 cup shredded lettuce
- 1 tbsp lime juice
- 1 tsp chili powder

Instructions:

1. Toast corn tortillas until crispy.
2. Spread mashed black beans over each tortilla and top with avocado slices.
3. Sprinkle with cheddar cheese, lettuce, lime juice, and chili powder.

Greek Spanakopita (Spinach Pie)

This Greek pastry combines flaky phyllo dough with a calcium-rich spinach and feta filling.

Ingredients:

- 2 cups fresh spinach, chopped (245 mg calcium)
- 1/2 cup crumbled feta cheese (200 mg calcium)
- 1/4 cup ricotta cheese (120 mg calcium)
- 1 clove garlic, minced
- 6 sheets phyllo dough
- 2 tbsp olive oil

Instructions:

1. Preheat oven to 375°F (190°C).
2. Sauté garlic and spinach until wilted. Let cool, then mix with feta and ricotta cheese.
3. Brush phyllo sheets with olive oil and layer them in a baking dish. Add the spinach mixture and fold the phyllo over to seal.
4. Bake for 25–30 minutes until golden and crispy.

West African Peanut Stew

A rich and creamy stew with calcium from peanuts and leafy greens.

Ingredients:

- 1 cup peanut butter (176 mg calcium)
- 2 cups chopped kale (177 mg calcium per cup)
- 1 sweet potato, diced (40 mg calcium)
- 1 can diced tomatoes
- 2 cups vegetable broth
- 1 clove garlic, minced
- 1 tsp paprika
- 1 tbsp olive oil
- Salt and pepper to taste

Instructions:

1. Heat olive oil in a pot and sauté the garlic. Add sweet potatoes and paprika and cook for 5 minutes.
2. Stir in tomatoes, peanut butter, and vegetable broth. Simmer until sweet potatoes are tender.
3. Add kale and cook until wilted. Season with salt and pepper before serving.

Italian White Bean and Kale Bruschetta

A flavorful Italian appetizer combining calcium-rich beans and kale.

Ingredients:

- 1 can white beans, drained and rinsed (100 mg calcium)
- 2 cups kale, chopped (177 mg calcium)
- 1 clove garlic, minced
- 1 tbsp olive oil
- 4 slices whole-grain bread
- 1 tbsp balsamic vinegar

Instructions:

1. Heat olive oil in a pan and sauté garlic. Add kale and cook until wilted.
2. Stir in white beans and balsamic vinegar. Cook for 2–3 minutes.
3. Toast bread slices and top with the bean and kale mixture. Serve warm.

Korean Kimchi Fried Rice

This Korean dish combines tangy kimchi with calcium-rich sesame seeds and greens.

Ingredients:

- 2 cups cooked brown rice
- 1/2 cup kimchi, chopped
- 1/2 cup spinach, chopped (60 mg calcium)
- 1 tbsp sesame oil
- 1 tbsp soy sauce (low sodium)
- 1 tbsp sesame seeds (88 mg calcium)
- 1 egg (optional, for topping)

Instructions:

1. Heat sesame oil in a skillet over medium heat. Add kimchi and cook for 2 minutes.
2. Stir in rice, spinach, and soy sauce. Cook until heated through.
3. Sprinkle with sesame seeds and top with a fried egg, if desired.

Ensure meals include a balance of protein, carbohydrates, and healthy fats, along with essential nutrients for bone health.

Supplements can help when dietary intake is insufficient, especially for those with dietary restrictions. Choose high-quality supplements that provide clear information about dosage and ingredients. It's recommended that adults get 1,000–1,200 mg of calcium and 600–800 IU of vitamin D daily. Always consult your healthcare provider before starting new supplements to avoid potential interactions with medications.

Research shows that calcium and vitamin D supplementation effectively reduce fracture risk, especially in older adults. However, experts emphasize that nutrients from food are generally more beneficial than supplements, as they contain additional nutrients that work synergistically to improve health.

Chapter 5: Exercise and Mobility

Imagine standing at the edge of a beautiful forest, excited to explore the winding trails ahead, but a small voice inside you whispers, "What if you fall?" This fear of fractures can turn even the simplest activities into daunting challenges when living with osteoporosis. It's natural to feel hesitant, but the good news is that exercise is one of the most powerful tools available to help strengthen your bones, boost your overall health, and regain the confidence to live a full and active life.

Gaining confidence through exercise doesn't happen overnight, but with a well-structured, consistent routine, you'll begin to notice improvements in both your physical strength and your mental resilience. Each small victory—whether it's walking a little farther or standing a little taller—helps break the cycle of fear, allowing you to engage with the world around you without constant anxiety about fractures or falls.

The Importance of Physical Activity

Exercise is critical for maintaining bone health, acting like a natural medicine for your bones. Weight-bearing and resistance exercises stimulate bone growth by putting stress on your bones, prompting them to grow denser and stronger. This process, known as stress-induced bone growth, is essential for preserving bone density and slowing the progression of osteoporosis. As you lift weights, your muscles become stronger to handle the load. Similarly, when you engage in weight-bearing exercises, your bones adapt to stress, reducing the risk of fractures.

Beyond bone health, regular physical activity offers numerous other benefits. Improved cardiovascular health lowers the risk of heart disease, and stronger muscles support and protect bones in daily activities. Exercises that improve balance and coordination, like yoga and Tai Chi, are particularly valuable because they reduce the risk of falls, a major concern for osteoporosis patients.

Getting started with exercise can be intimidating, especially if you're worried about injury. The key is to begin gently and build your strength over time. Low-impact exercises such as walking, swimming, or cycling are excellent starting points because they improve cardiovascular fitness while being easy on the joints and bones. Incorporating flexibility exercises like stretching or yoga into your routine will also help you avoid stiffness and maintain a full range of motion, which is essential for mobility.

To stay motivated, set realistic goals. For instance, start walking for 20 minutes three times a week and gradually increase the duration and frequency as you build endurance. An exercise partner can also keep you accountable and make the experience more enjoyable. Logging your workouts in a journal or app allows you to track your progress and see how far you've come, which can be encouraging when motivation dips.

Remember, consistency is key. Exercise for bone health is a long-term commitment, not a quick fix. Find activities you enjoy, whether it's dancing, yoga, or gardening, and stick with them. The more you move, the more your bones will benefit.

Weight-Bearing Exercises Explained

Weight-bearing exercises are the foundation of maintaining bone strength. These activities require your bones to support your body weight and work against gravity, which encourages your bones to become stronger and denser. There are two types of weight-bearing exercises: high-impact and low-impact.

High-impact exercises include activities like running, jumping, or dancing. These exercises are highly effective for building bone density but may not be suitable for everyone, especially those with advanced osteoporosis or joint issues. For many, low-impact exercises such as walking, hiking, or using an elliptical machine provide similar benefits without the risk of injury.

One of the simplest and most effective weight-bearing exercises is walking. Walking at a brisk pace promotes bone health without requiring special equipment or a gym membership. You can walk outdoors on a treadmill or even indoors at home. Hiking offers an additional challenge by incorporating varied terrains, which engage different muscles and stimulate bone growth in the lower body. Dancing is another enjoyable weight-bearing activity that combines fun with fitness—whether you prefer ballroom, salsa, or freestyle dancing in your living room, you're building bone density while improving coordination.

As with any exercise, proper technique is essential. Ensure you maintain good posture while walking or hiking: keep your shoulders back, head up, and arms swinging naturally. Wear supportive shoes to absorb impact and protect your joints. Starting with a five-minute warm-up and ending with a cool-down stretch will help prevent injury and ease muscle tension.

For those who need extra support or have mobility concerns, walking poles can offer stability and distribute body weight more evenly, reducing strain on your bones and joints. If you prefer exercising indoors, an elliptical machine provides a low-impact, joint-friendly alternative that still challenges your bones. You can adjust the resistance and incline as you build strength, making this a versatile tool for weight-bearing exercise.

Balance and Coordination Training

Balance and coordination are crucial, especially for those with osteoporosis, as they help prevent falls, which can lead to fractures. Strong stabilizing muscles and improved proprioception—the body's ability to sense its position in space—are key to maintaining balance and preventing injuries. Incorporating targeted balance exercises into your routine can enhance your stability and confidence in daily activities.

Begin with simple exercises like standing on one leg. This may sound easy, but it engages your stabilizing muscles, improving balance over time. Stand near a sturdy surface, like a chair or countertop, for support. Shift your weight onto one leg and lift the other leg slightly off the ground. Hold this position for 10 seconds or longer, depending on your ability. As you progress, try balancing without assistance and aim to increase your hold time gradually. To make the exercise more challenging, incorporate dynamic movements like lifting and lowering the raised leg or extending it forward or backward.

Another excellent balance exercise is the heel-to-toe walk. Imagine walking in a straight line, placing the heel of one foot directly in front of the toes of the other foot. This exercise mimics walking on a balance beam and strengthens both balance and coordination. Focus on controlled, slow movements to ensure proper technique. To increase difficulty, try walking backward or closing your eyes briefly (only if it's safe to do so).

Consider Tai Chi, which combines slow, flowing movements with focused breathing for a more holistic approach. Tai Chi is particularly beneficial for balance, coordination, and mental focus, making it ideal for individuals with osteoporosis. Its low-impact nature reduces the risk of strain or injury and can be adapted to suit any fitness level. Regular practice has been shown to enhance proprioception, improve posture, and increase lower-body strength. Tai Chi sessions often include movements like the "single whip" and "brush knee," which gently challenge balance and flexibility.

If Tai Chi doesn't resonate, other options like yoga or Pilates offer similar benefits. Yoga poses like the tree pose or Warrior III emphasize balance, while Pilates strengthens the core, a crucial stability component. These practices build physical strength and improve mindfulness, helping you feel more grounded and in control.

Balance training can also be incorporated into daily activities. For example, brushing your teeth while standing on one leg or walking slowly while carrying a light object can engage your stabilizing muscles. Even small adjustments to your routine, like taking stairs instead of elevators, help enhance coordination and balance over time.

By dedicating 10–15 minutes daily to balance and coordination exercises, you can significantly reduce your risk of falls, improve your overall stability, and enhance your quality of life. Small, consistent efforts lead to meaningful progress, empowering you to navigate daily activities confidently.

Safe and Effective Strength Training

Strength training is another critical component of osteoporosis management. By building muscle strength, you create a support system for your bones, reducing their load during everyday movements. This not only helps prevent fractures but also enhances mobility and independence.

There are many ways to engage in strength training safely. Resistance bands are versatile tools that allow you to adjust the intensity of your workout. Exercises like bicep curls, leg lifts, and shoulder presses can easily be performed with resistance bands at home. Bodyweight exercises like squats and push-ups are also effective and can be done anywhere. Start with modified versions if needed, and gradually increase intensity as you build strength.

When using weights, begin with light dumbbells and focus on proper form. For example, keep your feet shoulder-width apart, back straight, and knees aligned with your toes when doing squats. To protect your joints, avoid letting your knees move past your toes. Push-ups, whether performed on your knees or a wall, help strengthen your upper body without overloading your bones.

The key to safe strength training is gradual progression. Start with lower resistance or lighter weights and increase as you become stronger. Always listen to your body and take breaks if you experience pain or discomfort.

Yoga and Pilates offer a unique blend of strength, flexibility, and balance training, making them ideal for people with osteoporosis. These practices improve core strength, supporting the spine and enhancing stability, while increasing joint flexibility and range of motion.

In Yoga, the Tree Pose improves balance and strengthens the legs. In this pose, you stand on one leg, with the other foot resting on your inner thigh or calf. It's a simple yet effective way to build strength while enhancing focus and concentration. Pilates, on the other hand, focuses on core stability and controlled movements. Exercises like the Bridge Pose strengthen the glutes, hamstrings, and lower back, all of which are important for supporting the spine and pelvis.

Both Yoga and Pilates incorporate mindfulness and controlled breathing, helping reduce stress—a key factor in managing osteoporosis. Stress increases cortisol levels, which can negatively impact bone health, so these practices offer both physical and mental benefits.

The Warrior pose builds leg strength and enhances balance. Move one foot back, bend the front knee and stretch your arms overhead. The Bridge pose supports the back and glutes while stretching the chest and spine. Rest on your back with your knees bent and feet flat on the floor, and raise your hips towards the roof. In Pilates, pelvic tilts support the lower back and abdominal muscles. Lie on your back with your knees bent and feet resting on the floor, and slowly tilt your pelvis upward. Leg circles boost hip mobility and strengthen the core. Lie on your back with one leg raised towards the roof and make small, controlled circles. The modified plank supports the core and upper body. Start on your hands and knees, then extend one leg at a time to form a straight line from your head to your heels, maintaining the position while engaging your core.

Safety Adaptations in Yoga and Pilates

When practicing yoga or Pilates, safety is key to preventing injury and ensuring you're reaping the benefits without putting undue stress on your bones. Yoga props, such as blocks, straps, and bolsters, can be incredibly helpful for those with osteoporosis, as they allow you to maintain proper alignment and modify poses to suit your ability level.

For example, in the Tree Pose, where you stand on one leg to improve balance, you can place a yoga block under your hand for additional support. This stabilizes you as you improve your balance without the risk of falling. Straps can also be beneficial in poses like Seated Forward Bend, where they help you reach your feet without straining your back. These simple tools ensure you get the most out of your yoga practice while staying safe.

However, it's essential to avoid certain poses that can put too much stress on your spine, particularly deep twists, forward bends, or any exercise that involves rounding the back. These movements can compress the vertebrae and increase the risk of fractures. Instead, focus on gentle, controlled movements that build strength and stability, such as seated poses or standing postures with modifications.

Luckily, many resources are available to help you safely begin yoga and Pilates, even if you're new to exercise. Look for programs designed specifically for osteoporosis that provide clear instructions and modifications for various poses. Online platforms can offer Yoga and Pilates, beginner-friendly classes designed with osteoporosis in mind. By choosing the right resources and making adjustments, yoga and Pilates can become an integral part of your exercise routine, helping to improve flexibility, strength, and balance while protecting your bones.

Creating a Personalized Exercise Plan

A personalized exercise plan tailored to your fitness level and goals can be transformative in managing osteoporosis. The first step in developing your plan is assessing your fitness level. Consider any physical limitations, past injuries, or health concerns that might impact your ability to exercise. For example, if you've recently recovered from a fracture or surgery, your plan should start with low-impact activities to avoid putting stress on weakened bones. Consulting a healthcare provider or physical therapist can also provide valuable insight into what exercises are safe and beneficial for your condition.

Once you clearly understand your starting point, it's time to set realistic, achievable goals. Setting specific, measurable goals will keep you focused and motivated. Instead of simply saying, "I want to exercise more," try a goal like, "I will walk for 20 minutes, three times a week," or, "I will complete 10 minutes of balance exercises every morning." Goals like these are clear, trackable, and flexible, allowing you to celebrate progress and make adjustments as needed.

Incorporating different types of exercises into your plan is also essential. A well-rounded plan includes weight-bearing exercises for bone health, such as walking, dancing, or stair climbing. Balance exercises, like standing on one leg or practicing Tai Chi, are crucial for reducing the risk of falls, while strength training with resistance bands or light weights builds muscle to support your bones. Flexibility exercises, like yoga or gentle stretching, enhance mobility and help maintain a full range of motion. Variety not only ensures that you're working on all areas of fitness but also keeps your routine engaging and prevents overuse injuries that can result from repeatedly doing the same type of exercise.

To stay consistent, schedule your workouts as part of your daily routine. Consider joining a class or finding an exercise buddy to make the experience more enjoyable and hold yourself accountable. With a personalized plan that suits your needs and preferences, managing osteoporosis becomes a proactive and empowering part of your lifestyle.

Your Personal Movement Journey

Navigating exercise with osteoporosis isn't about pushing limits—it's about understanding your body and moving smartly. This chapter is your roadmap to creating a sustainable, safe, and effective exercise routine that supports your bone health and overall well-being.

Myth-Busting: Exercise and Osteoporosis

Common misconceptions can prevent people from achieving optimal health. Let's address some prevalent myths:

- **Myth**: Exercise is too risky with osteoporosis
- **Reality**: Targeted, appropriate exercise is one of the most powerful tools for managing bone health
- **Myth**: You're too old to start exercising
- **Reality**: It's never too late to improve strength, balance, and bone density

Practical Exercise Planning: A Step-by-Step Guide

Step 1: Professional Consultation

Before beginning any exercise program:

- Schedule a comprehensive medical assessment
- Discuss your specific bone density measurements
- Get personalized recommendations from:
  - Your primary care physician
  - Endocrinologist
  - Physical therapist specializing in bone health
  - Certified osteoporosis fitness trainer

What to Discuss in Your Consultation

- Current bone density status
- Fracture history
- Medication interactions
- Existing mobility limitations
- Personal fitness goals

Step 2: Assessing Your Current Fitness Level

Self-Assessment Checklist

1. Can you stand on one leg for 10 seconds?

2. Do you experience pain during light activities?

3. How many stairs can you climb without resting?

4. Can you sit and stand from a chair without using your hands?

Pro Tip: Don't get discouraged by current limitations. These are starting points, not finish lines.

Step 3: Creating Your Personalized Exercise Toolkit

Equipment Recommendations

Budget-Friendly Options:

- Resistance bands ($10-$20)
- Yoga mat ($15-$30)
- Light dumbbells (2-5 lbs)
- Stability ball
- Comfortable, supportive shoes

Home Exercise Space

- Clear, open area
- Non-slip flooring
- Nearby chair for support
- Good lighting
- Water bottle
- Optional: Full-length mirror

Step 4: Building Your Weekly Exercise Routine

Beginner's Weekly Template

Monday: Balance and Flexibility

- 15-minute gentle yoga
- 10-minute balance exercises
- Stretching

Tuesday: Strength Training

- Resistance band exercises

- Light dumbbell work
- Chair-supported movements

Wednesday: Rest and Recovery

- Gentle walking
- Light stretching
- Deep breathing exercises

Thursday: Cardiovascular Health

- 30-minute walking
- Low-impact dancing
- Swimming (if available)

Friday: Strength and Balance

- Repeated Tuesday's routine
- Add new variations

Saturday: Enjoyable Movement

- Gardening
- Gentle hiking
- Social dance class

Sunday: Active Recovery

- Stretching
- Meditation
- Light walking

Progression Strategies

Beginner Level (0-3 Months)

- Focus on form and consistency
- Use support (chairs, walls)
- Start with 10-15 minute sessions
- Prioritize safety over intensity

Intermediate Level (3-6 Months)

- Increase session duration
- Add light weights
- Introduce more complex movements
- Improve balance challenges

Advanced Level (6-12 Months)

- Implement progressive resistance
- Try group fitness classes
- Explore more dynamic exercises
- Work with specialized trainer

Safety Red Flags: When to Stop

Immediately cease exercise and consult your healthcare provider if you experience:

- Sharp, stabbing pain
- Sudden weakness
- Dizziness
- Chest discomfort
- Unusual fatigue
- Breathing difficulties

Technology and Exercise Support

Recommended Apps

- Silver Sneakers
- Fitbit Senior Fitness
- AARP Fitness App
- Yoga for Seniors
- Balance Training Platforms

Tracking Progress

- Take monthly measurements
- Photograph exercise forms
- Keep a mobility journal
- Note energy levels and mood changes

Psychological Aspects of Exercise

Motivation Techniques

- Set small, achievable goals
- Celebrate every milestone
- Join support groups
- Share your journey with family
- Be kind to yourself

Mental Health Benefits

- Reduced anxiety
- Improved self-confidence
- Enhanced social connections
- Sense of empowerment
- Stress reduction

Your Movement, Your Power

Exercise with osteoporosis isn't about perfection—it's about progression. Each movement celebrates what your body can do, not a punishment for what it can't.

Remember: You're not just exercising to prevent bone loss. You're building strength, confidence, and a vibrant life.

Recommended Resources

- Local osteoporosis support groups
- Senior fitness centers
- Online exercise communities

- Certified osteoporosis fitness trainers

Staying Motivated and Consistent

Sticking to an exercise plan can be difficult, but there are ways to stay motivated. Keeping an exercise journal is a great strategy for tracking progress and reflecting on your achievements. Write down your workouts, how you felt before and after, and any improvements you notice. This record can be a powerful motivator when you look back and see how far you've come.

Celebrating small milestones is another excellent way to stay engaged with your routine. Whether it's walking an extra five minutes or lifting a heavier weight, these achievements are worth celebrating. Reward yourself with something enjoyable, like new workout gear or a relaxing activity, to keep your motivation high.

Joining an exercise group or class can also be incredibly helpful. Exercising with others who share similar goals provides accountability and support. Look for community or online classes designed for individuals with osteoporosis. These classes often include modifications for all fitness levels and are led by instructors who understand the unique needs of people with bone health concerns.

As we wrap up this chapter, remember that a personalized and consistent exercise routine is one of the most powerful tools for managing osteoporosis. Combining weight-bearing exercises, balance training, and strength workouts can support your bones, improve mobility, and protect yourself from fractures. With safety adaptations like yoga props and personalized modifications, you can exercise confidently, knowing you're minimizing risks.

Exercise is not just about physical health; it also boosts mental well-being and enhances quality of life. As you embark on this journey, remember that consistency, patience, and enjoyment are the keys to success. With a well-rounded approach and a commitment to staying active, you'll be well on your way to stronger bones and a more vibrant, active life.

In the next chapter, we'll explore how to create a safe home environment that further reduces the risk of falls and injuries, ensuring that you continue to live independently and confidently.

Chapter 6: Preventing Falls and Injuries

Imagine relaxing in your cozy living room, enjoying a cup of tea, when you notice your favorite rug bunched at the edge. It's a small thing, easy to overlook, but in that moment, you realize it could be dangerous. You've heard stories of people tripping and falling, and with osteoporosis, the risk is even higher. A simple stumble could lead to a serious fracture. Suddenly, what was once a comfortable home begins to feel like a source of anxiety. But it doesn't have to be this way. By making a few thoughtful adjustments, you can transform your home into a safe space that reduces the risk of falls, ensuring you feel secure in every room.

Home Safety Modifications

Common household hazards are often hidden in plain sight, presenting risks we might not immediately notice. Loose rugs and carpets, for example, can easily slip or bunch up, turning into tripping hazards. Picture yourself walking through the living room; your foot catches on the corner of a rug, and suddenly, you're on the floor. Another risky area is cluttered walkways. Shoes, magazines, and electrical cords left in the path can create unnecessary dangers. Then there's the bathroom—wet, slippery floors from showers or sinks are particularly hazardous for falls.

To address these risks, start by securing loose rugs with non-slip pads. These pads grip the floor, keeping rugs in place and reducing the chance of them shifting. For carpets, ensure they're firmly attached to the floor. Consider replacing high-pile rugs with low-pile options that are less likely to catch your feet, reducing the risk further.

Clearing clutter from walkways is another simple but essential step. Designate a space for shoes near the entrance, use cable organizers to manage electrical cords, and ensure that items like magazines have a proper place. Consider creating designated "no-clutter zones" in high-traffic areas, such as hallways, doorways, and near staircases, where tripping risks are higher.

Proper lighting is another key factor in preventing falls. Hallways, staircases, and frequently used rooms should be well-lit, with bright, energy-efficient bulbs providing consistent illumination. Motion-sensor night lights are an excellent addition, as they turn on automatically when movement is detected, guiding you safely through your home at night. Smart lighting systems can allow you to control brightness and timing with voice commands or a smartphone app, ensuring you never walk into a dark room. Use light switches that are easily accessible and glow in the dark for added convenience.

Fall-Proofing Your Living Space

Each room in your home presents unique challenges, but with a few strategic changes, you can dramatically reduce your fall risk. Let's take a closer look at key rooms in the home:

- **Kitchen**: Keep frequently used items within easy reach to avoid unnecessary stretching or climbing. Store heavy or bulky objects at waist height to reduce strain. Use non-slip mats near the sink and stove for added stability. Avoid standing on chairs or unstable stools to reach high shelves—use a sturdy step stool with a handrail instead. Consider rearranging items periodically to ensure your kitchen remains accessible as your needs evolve.

- **Bedroom**: Position your nightstand close to the bed for easy access to essentials like glasses, medication, and phones. Use a lamp with a touch sensor or an easy-to-reach switch for nighttime visibility. Ensure the area around your bed is free from loose mats or cords that could trip you. Bed risers can make getting in and out of bed easier, and adjustable beds may provide additional comfort and safety. Motion-activated lights under the bed can softly illuminate the floor, guiding your steps during nighttime trips.

- **Living Room**: Arrange furniture to create clear, open walkways, avoiding low tables or footstools that could obstruct your path. If you have a coffee table, make sure it's sturdy with rounded corners to prevent injuries if you bump into it. Secure any loose cords from electronic devices using cable organizers. Replace unstable or wobbly furniture with more secure options.

Assistive Devices and Technology

For those with osteoporosis, assistive devices can be crucial in enhancing safety and independence. Common devices like canes and walkers provide essential stability, allowing you to confidently move around. Grab bars and handrails in key locations, such as the bathroom and stairways, offer extra support when standing up or navigating tricky spaces. Reachers and grabbers are another useful tool, allowing you to pick up objects without needing to bend over.

Technology has also provided us with new ways to stay safe. Fall detection devices can automatically sense a fall and alert emergency contacts, while smart home systems let you control lights, thermostats, and alarms using voice commands or mobile apps. These technologies can provide added peace of mind and convenience.

When choosing assistive devices, consult with your healthcare provider to ensure you select the right tools for your specific needs. Proper fitting is essential for canes and walkers—your elbow should be slightly bent when you hold the handle. Grab bars must be securely installed into wall studs for maximum stability.

Regular maintenance of assistive devices is crucial. For canes and walkers, check for wear on rubber tips and replace them as needed. For smart devices, keep the software updated to ensure proper functioning.

Safe Movement and Daily Activities

Everyday movements like getting in and out of bed or standing up from a chair require extra attention when you have osteoporosis. To get out of bed safely, start by sitting on the edge with your feet flat on the floor, then use your hands to push yourself into a standing position. When sitting down or standing up from a chair, use the armrests for support, and always move slowly to maintain your balance.

Stairs are another common area of concern. Always use handrails for support, and take your time, placing your whole foot on each step before moving to the next. Shoes with non-slip soles are essential for indoor and outdoor activities, providing extra traction and reducing the risk of slipping.

Emergency Preparedness for Falls

While we take every precaution to prevent falls, it's essential to be prepared in case they do happen. Keep emergency contacts easily accessible in several locations around your home. Having a phone within reach at all times is crucial, whether it's a cell phone, cordless phone, or medical alert system.

Learning how to get up safely after a fall is also important. If you can, roll onto your side, then use your hands and knees to crawl to a sturdy piece of furniture, such as a chair, to help yourself stand. If you cannot get up, use your phone or medical alert device to call for help.

Importance of Routine Vision and Hearing Checks

Good vision and hearing play a critical role in fall prevention. Poor eyesight can make it difficult to detect obstacles, and hearing impairments might prevent you from noticing hazards like a family member calling out a warning or the sound of an approaching object. Regular check-ups with an optometrist and audiologist can ensure your senses are sharp, reducing the likelihood of accidents. Update your prescription glasses if needed, and consider wearing hearing aids if recommended.

Practicing Mindful Movement

Mindfulness isn't just for relaxation—it can help prevent falls, too. Moving with intention makes you more likely to notice potential hazards and maintain your balance. For example:

- Always look ahead while walking instead of focusing on the ground.
- Pause before transitioning positions, such as standing up from a chair or bed.
- Avoid rushing, particularly on stairs or uneven surfaces.

In the next chapter, we will discuss the importance of emotional support and well-being.

Chapter 7: Emotional Well-being and Support

Imagine yourself sitting in your doctor's office, heart racing as you await your latest bone density test results. The doctor enters, sits down, and speaks the words you've dreaded: "You have osteoporosis." Suddenly, a wave of emotions hits—shock, denial, and fear of the future. This chapter delves into handling these emotions and discovering how to thrive emotionally while living with osteoporosis.

The initial emotional response to an osteoporosis diagnosis can be overwhelming. Feelings of shock, denial, or fear about the future are normal. It's difficult to accept that your bones aren't as strong as they once were, especially if you've led an active life. Thoughts like, *This can't be happening to me* or doubts about the diagnosis may flood your mind. Taking time to process the news is essential.

Concerns about future health, fractures, or lifestyle changes can create anxiety. Activities you once enjoyed may now seem risky, and you may wonder how to adjust. While these worries can feel overwhelming, know that many people continue to live fulfilling lives with osteoporosis.

Journaling can be an excellent way to process these emotions. Writing your thoughts down provides clarity, helping you manage worries. Talking to a trusted friend or family member can also offer emotional support. Simply knowing someone is listening can make a significant difference.

If you need deeper emotional guidance, seeking professional counseling may help. A therapist can help you work through complicated feelings and build resilience. A healthcare provider or local resources can help you find a counselor who specializes in chronic illness.

Be kind to yourself during this time. Avoid self-blame, as osteoporosis is influenced by many factors outside your control. Self-care practices—whether a warm bath, reading, or spending time outdoors—can be small yet meaningful acts of self-kindness. Mindfulness and breathing exercises also help ease anxiety, grounding you in the present.

Hobbies and activities you love can also offer a sense of normalcy. Whether playing an instrument, gardening, or painting, these moments of joy remind you that osteoporosis doesn't define your life.

Reflection Section: Self-Compassion Practice

Take a moment to reflect on the activities that bring you joy and peace. List three self-care activities that you genuinely enjoy—whether it's reading a book, taking a warm bath, or going for a walk in nature—and commit to incorporating them into your weekly routine. These activities may seem simple, but they are essential in maintaining your emotional well-being and helping you manage the challenges of osteoporosis.

Remember, self-care isn't indulgent; it's an act of kindness toward yourself, a way to recharge and restore balance in your life. These small but meaningful moments help reduce stress, foster a positive mindset, and remind you that caring for yourself is just as important as any medical treatment. By consistently carving out time for self-care, you nurture your mental and emotional resilience, which in turn supports your physical health and overall quality of life.

Consider setting reminders or scheduling these moments into your week—just as you would with any important appointment. Taking this time for yourself is not a luxury; it is vital in sustaining your energy, focus, and well-being as you navigate your osteoporosis journey.

Building a Support Network

An osteoporosis diagnosis can initially feel isolating, but building a strong support network can lighten the load. Social support is crucial for emotional well-being. When surrounded by people who understand your journey, the burden of managing osteoporosis feels lighter.

Begin with family and friends. Often, loved ones want to help but aren't sure how. Have an honest conversation about your needs—whether it's attending doctor visits, running errands, or simply offering a listening ear. Don't hesitate to ask for specific support.

Community groups, either local or virtual, provide an excellent opportunity to connect with others who understand what you're going through. Look for osteoporosis support groups or chronic illness groups through hospitals or community centers. These spaces offer shared experiences, valuable advice, and emotional support.

In today's digital age, online communities are a valuable resource. Online platforms, forums, and support apps offer a chance to connect with people worldwide, providing comfort and encouragement. These spaces can be helpful if you prefer sharing anonymously or need advice on managing symptoms, treatment options, or emotional challenges.

Healthcare professionals also play a vital role in your support network. Regular check-ins with your doctor can help you stay on top of your treatment plan. At the same time, mental health professionals can offer tools to manage anxiety or depression related to osteoporosis. A physical therapist can help with mobility, and a nutritionist can guide your dietary needs.

Assertive communication is key to maintaining a strong support network. Be clear about how you're feeling and what type of support you need. Specific requests, such as asking for help with grocery shopping or needing to talk, make it easier for others to provide meaningful help. And remember to express gratitude—small gestures of appreciation go a long way in nurturing relationships.

Interactive Element: Support Network Checklist

Take a few moments to create a list of people you can rely on for support in your life. Think about family members, close friends, healthcare professionals, and community resources that can offer help during your osteoporosis journey. These individuals can provide emotional comfort, practical assistance, or expert guidance as you manage your condition. Remember, you don't have to face osteoporosis alone—your support network is there to lift you up when needed.

Consider expanding your network by reaching out to someone new, whether it's a healthcare provider you haven't consulted yet, a local support group, or even a trusted neighbor. Growing your circle of support can provide fresh perspectives, new ideas, and different types of assistance you may not have considered before. A broader network gives you access to more resources, advice, and encouragement, which are crucial in maintaining your physical and emotional well-being.

As you create this list, reflect on each person's value to your life. Whether they provide a listening ear, medical expertise, or companionship, their role is essential in helping you navigate osteoporosis confidently. Keep this list handy, and don't hesitate to lean on your support system—asking for help when needed is a sign of strength, not weakness.

The Role of Mental Health in Physical Health

Mental and physical health are closely linked, especially when managing a condition like osteoporosis. Stress triggers the release of cortisol, a hormone that, when elevated, can weaken bones by increasing bone resorption and slowing bone formation. Prolonged stress can accelerate bone loss, worsening osteoporosis. Conversely, a positive mental state can enhance your body's ability to heal and maintain health. Feeling mentally strong makes you more likely to engage in beneficial activities like exercising, eating well, and staying social.

Effectively managing stress is essential. Begin by identifying your stress triggers, which may include daily frustrations or larger worries, such as financial concerns or health anxieties. Once you pinpoint what's causing stress, you can create strategies to manage it. Simple relaxation techniques, such as deep breathing or progressive muscle relaxation, can be powerful tools for calming the mind and body.

Living with osteoporosis can also bring specific mental health challenges like anxiety or depression, often fueled by the fear of fractures or loss of independence. Recognizing these emotional difficulties early on is key to managing them. Resources like mental health hotlines, counseling services, and online therapy platforms offer support when needed. Apps like Headspace and Calm can also guide you through mindfulness exercises to help reduce stress and improve emotional well-being.

Resource List: Mental Health Resources

- National Alliance on Mental Illness (NAMI) Helpline
- Headspace (Mindfulness and meditation app)
- BetterHelp (Online counseling platform)

Planning for Long-Term Health

Managing osteoporosis is a long-term commitment. Setting realistic health goals—whether maintaining bone density or enhancing mobility—provides direction. Regular checkups, bone density tests, and a flexible approach to treatment and lifestyle will keep you on track.

Make dietary and exercise changes as part of a sustainable lifestyle, ensuring you get enough calcium and vitamin D, remain physically active, and avoid smoking or excessive drinking habits. Use resources such as support groups, healthcare professionals, and online forums to stay Dietary and exercise changes are part of a sustainable lifestyle.

Resource List: Ongoing Support

- Bone Health and Osteoporosis Foundation
- Mayo Clinic
- Local osteoporosis support groups

Celebrating Progress and Setting Future Goals

Recognizing your progress is vital. Whether it's sticking to an exercise routine or seeing an improvement in bone density, acknowledging these milestones helps sustain motivation. Reward yourself with simple joys, like a special outing, sharing progress with loved ones, or reflecting in your journal.

Set new goals to keep pushing forward—whether it's trying a new exercise, joining a support group, or improving your diet. Stay adaptable and celebrate even the smallest victories, as they contribute to your overall success in managing osteoporosis.

Interactive Element: Milestone Celebration Ideas

- Plan a special outing
- Share progress with friends or family
- Reflect on personal growth in a journal

Chapter 8: Staying Informed and Engaged

Picture yourself in your favorite chair, skimming through a magazine, when an article about a breakthrough osteoporosis treatment catches your eye. Your heart races. Could this be the solution you've been seeking? Staying up to date with the latest research and advancements isn't just interesting—it's essential for managing osteoporosis. In a rapidly evolving medical landscape, staying informed can significantly improve your quality of life.

Keeping up with osteoporosis research is more than just being aware of treatment options—it's about empowering yourself to make decisions that align with your evolving health needs. The landscape of osteoporosis management is constantly changing, with new therapies and technological innovations introduced regularly. As patients become more proactive in their care, having a finger on the pulse of research can help you be part of the conversation with your healthcare team, ensuring that your treatment plan is the best available.

Advancements in the field of biotechnology and genetic research are opening new doors for osteoporosis treatment. Researchers are now exploring the role of genetic predisposition to osteoporosis, which may one day lead to personalized treatments based on your DNA. Imagine having access to therapies tailored specifically to your genetic makeup, potentially increasing effectiveness and reducing side effects. Keeping an eye on these developments through trustworthy medical sources can provide you with exciting insights into the future of bone health.

In addition, regenerative medicine is an emerging area of interest in osteoporosis treatment. Stem cell research explores the potential to regenerate damaged bone tissue, offering hope for those with severe osteoporosis. While still in the early stages, clinical trials are underway, and future breakthroughs in this area could drastically change the treatment landscape. Awareness of these pioneering developments might allow you to explore participation in relevant clinical trials or adopt newer therapies as they become available.

Technology is also revolutionizing the way osteoporosis is diagnosed and monitored. Artificial intelligence (AI) in analyzing bone density scans improves the precision of osteoporosis diagnosis. AI algorithms can detect minute changes in bone structure that may be missed by the human eye, leading to earlier interventions and personalized treatment plans. Staying updated with these technological advancements can empower you to ask your healthcare provider about the possibility of incorporating such innovative tools into your care.

Interactive Element: Research Spotlight

- **Biotechnology and Genetics:** Stay informed about genetic predisposition research.

- **Stem Cell Therapies:** Learn about regenerative medicine and clinical trials.

- **AI in Diagnostics:** Explore how artificial intelligence is transforming osteoporosis diagnosis.

Advocacy and Raising Awareness

Beyond staying informed for personal benefit, advocating for osteoporosis awareness can bring about meaningful change. Advocacy doesn't just happen at the government or policy level—it can happen in your community, workplace, or social circles. You have the power to raise awareness, reduce stigma, and promote education about osteoporosis.

Many individuals feel isolated after a diagnosis, but by sharing your story and experiences, you can help others understand that osteoporosis is manageable. Speaking at local health events or writing articles for community newsletters can spread awareness about early detection, lifestyle changes, and available resources. For example, many people don't know that osteoporosis can affect individuals as young as their 30s due to genetic factors or other underlying conditions. Your voice can help highlight that osteoporosis is not just an "older person's disease."

You could also consider advocating for policy changes. Numerous global and national organizations, such as the Bone Health and Osteoporosis Foundation (BHOF) and the International Osteoporosis Foundation (IOF), promote better healthcare policies for osteoporosis screening and treatment. By joining these efforts, you can influence healthcare coverage to ensure more individuals have access to diagnostic screenings and treatments at an affordable rate. Advocacy can include signing petitions, writing to government representatives, or participating in osteoporosis awareness campaigns like World Osteoporosis Day.

Additionally, advocating for improved osteoporosis education in schools, workplaces, and communities can have long-lasting effects. Many people are unaware of the preventive steps they can take early in life, such as engaging in weight-bearing exercises and consuming adequate calcium and vitamin D. By pushing for more comprehensive osteoporosis education, particularly for younger audiences, you can help future generations take control of their bone health early on.

Exploring Cutting-Edge Treatments

The future of osteoporosis treatment holds exciting potential, and it's important to remain open to these innovations. For instance, biophosphonate alternatives are being explored as potential breakthroughs. Current treatments like biophosphonates can slow bone loss, but newer medications may offer more targeted action with fewer long-term side effects. The development of anabolic therapies, which promote bone formation rather than merely slowing its loss, represents a promising area of research.

Monoclonal antibodies are another emerging treatment for osteoporosis. These lab-made molecules can mimic the body's natural defenses and are being used to slow bone resorption while enhancing bone formation. Drugs like romosozumab, a monoclonal antibody, are at the forefront of these advancements. While newer, these treatments are gaining momentum as clinical trials demonstrate their effectiveness in reducing fracture risk.

In addition, hormone replacement therapies (HRT) are evolving, with new formulations being designed to reduce side effects and improve effectiveness. Post-menopausal women, for example, may benefit from these innovations, which can provide a safer alternative to traditional HRT options.

Staying aware of such cutting-edge treatments means you'll be prepared to discuss them with your doctor when they become widely available. Being proactive about incorporating new options into your treatment plan ensures you get the most advanced care possible.

Expanding Lifestyle Modifications Beyond Diet and Exercise

While diet and exercise are cornerstones of osteoporosis management, other, often overlooked lifestyle changes can support bone health. For example, improving your sleep hygiene can have a profound effect on bone metabolism. Studies show that poor sleep can interfere with your body's ability to repair itself, including bone regeneration. Aiming for 7-9 hours of quality sleep, practicing good sleep habits, and addressing issues like sleep apnea can contribute to better bone health.

Reducing stress is another important factor in osteoporosis management. Chronic stress leads to elevated cortisol levels, a hormone that can decrease bone density over time. Mindfulness practices, such as meditation, yoga, or tai chi, improve balance and flexibility and reduce stress, offering dual benefits for both your mind and bones.

Hydration is often underappreciated in the conversation about bone health. Staying hydrated helps your body maintain the right balance of minerals needed for bone density. Ensuring adequate water intake throughout the day supports overall health and enhances the effectiveness of other osteoporosis treatments.

Finally, managing comorbid conditions, such as diabetes or thyroid disorders, is critical. These conditions can affect bone health in complex ways. For instance, uncontrolled diabetes can contribute to bone fragility, and certain thyroid disorders can accelerate bone loss. By keeping these conditions in check through medication, lifestyle adjustments, and regular monitoring, you can help protect your bones.

The Role of Digital Health Tools

Incorporating digital health tools into your osteoporosis management routine is becoming increasingly common. Wearable devices like smartwatches and fitness trackers can track your daily activity, including steps, workouts, and sleep quality, providing valuable insights into your health. Some advanced devices even monitor your heart rate and stress levels, which can help you manage the impact of stress on your bones.

Virtual consultations and telemedicine have also transformed healthcare access. Now, you can consult with osteoporosis specialists from the comfort of your home, making staying engaged with your treatment plan easier without the hassle of in-person appointments. Many healthcare providers are embracing telemedicine as a convenient way to monitor your condition, adjust medications, and answer questions in real-time.

Interactive Element: Digital Tools and Telemedicine

- **Fitness Trackers:** Use wearable devices to monitor your physical activity and sleep quality.

- **Telemedicine:** Schedule virtual appointments with your healthcare team to stay connected.

- **Health Apps:** Explore apps for nutrition tracking, exercise planning, and medication management.

In the next chapter, we'll explore other medical conditions that can co-exist alongside osteoporosis.

Chapter 9: Osteoporosis and Coexisting Conditions

Living with osteoporosis often involves more than simply managing bone health. Many individuals with osteoporosis find themselves facing other health challenges, as certain diseases and conditions can increase the risk of developing osteoporosis or make its management more complex. Understanding these connections can help you and your healthcare provider create a comprehensive plan that supports your entire health picture, whether it's joint issues, digestive concerns, or chronic illnesses. In this chapter, we'll explore some of the most common conditions frequently accompanying osteoporosis, their impact on bone health, and practical strategies for managing them together.

Osteoarthritis (OA) and Osteoporosis: Managing Joint and Bone Health Together

Osteoarthritis (OA) is a common degenerative joint disorder that causes cartilage between bones to break down, leading to joint pain, stiffness, and limited mobility. While OA and osteoporosis are separate conditions, they often coexist, particularly in older adults, complicating physical activity. The pain from OA can make movement challenging, yet inactivity may worsen joint stiffness and accelerate bone density loss in people with osteoporosis.

To manage both conditions together, a tailored approach using low-impact, joint-friendly exercises can effectively promote joint and bone health without undue stress. Water-based activities, like swimming and water aerobics, provide resistance to build muscle and support joint stability while minimizing joint impact. Incorporating gentle strength training with resistance bands helps strengthen the muscles around joints, which reduces OA-related pain, improves stability, and helps prevent osteoporosis-related fractures. Anti-inflammatory foods, including turmeric, berries, and green tea, can further support OA pain management by reducing inflammation and enhancing bone health.

Working with a physical therapist experienced in joint and bone health can be invaluable. They can guide adaptive exercise routines and joint-sparing techniques—such as ergonomic grips or braces—that reduce joint strain and allow for safe, consistent activity. Complementary therapies like acupuncture and therapeutic massage can relieve pain without increasing bone fragility, making them effective for ongoing OA and osteoporosis management.

Rheumatoid Arthritis (RA) and Osteoporosis: Navigating Immune and Bone Health

Rheumatoid arthritis (RA) is an autoimmune disorder that causes joint inflammation, resulting in pain, swelling, and joint deformity over time. Individuals with RA face a higher risk of developing osteoporosis due to both inflammation-related bone loss and the use of corticosteroid medications, which can weaken bones.

Managing RA and osteoporosis together requires a careful balance of anti-inflammatory and bone-supportive practices. Low-impact exercises like cycling, swimming, and gentle stretching (such as yoga) can enhance mobility, reduce joint stiffness, and support bone strength without exacerbating inflammation. Anti-inflammatory diets rich in omega-3 fatty acids, found in fish and flaxseeds, and antioxidants from colorful vegetables can help reduce RA symptoms while promoting bone density.

A rheumatologist can work with a primary care physician to develop a medication plan that balances inflammation control with bone health preservation. Regularly monitoring bone density, especially when taking corticosteroids, is essential. Supplementing with calcium and vitamin D, alongside RA medications, supports bone health. Additionally, complementary therapies like acupuncture and low-impact Pilates can improve joint function, reduce pain, and provide a holistic approach to managing both RA and osteoporosis.

Type 2 Diabetes and Osteoporosis: Balancing Blood Sugar and Bone Health

Type 2 diabetes can increase the risk of osteoporosis due to factors such as higher blood sugar levels and diabetes medications that may impact bone health. Elevated blood sugar can damage bone tissue over time, while some diabetes medications may reduce calcium absorption, leading to increased bone fragility.

To manage both conditions, maintaining stable blood sugar levels while prioritizing bone health is crucial. A diet low in refined sugars and rich in whole grains, leafy greens, and lean proteins can provide sustained energy and support bone density. Weight-bearing exercises like walking and strength training improve insulin sensitivity, stabilize blood sugar, and promote bone growth.

Working closely with an endocrinologist can ensure that diabetes medications are optimized to reduce bone health risks. Regularly monitoring blood sugar levels and bone density enables more personalized treatment adjustments. Weight management, which is essential for blood sugar control, also benefits bone density. Combining diabetes management with osteoporosis-friendly practices, such as low-impact strength training and dietary supplementation, creates a balanced approach that effectively addresses both conditions.

Celiac Disease and Osteoporosis: Supporting Bone Health Through Diet

Celiac disease, an autoimmune disorder triggered by gluten, can significantly impact bone health due to nutrient malabsorption, especially of calcium and vitamin D. This malabsorption leads to a higher risk of osteoporosis, as the body struggles to absorb essential bone-supporting nutrients.

A strict gluten-free diet is fundamental for individuals with both celiac disease and osteoporosis. Nutrient-rich gluten-free grains, like quinoa and brown rice, along with leafy greens and fortified gluten-free products, can provide essential vitamins and minerals. Calcium and vitamin D supplementation may be necessary to ensure bone health, as individuals with celiac disease often have low levels of these nutrients due to absorption issues.

Regular consultations with a dietitian specializing in celiac disease can help monitor nutrient levels and ensure a balanced gluten-free diet that meets bone health requirements. Weight-bearing and strength exercises, such as yoga and resistance band workouts, can further support bone density without causing gastrointestinal distress. Regular monitoring of bone density is also essential to assess the effectiveness of dietary and lifestyle interventions.

Chronic Kidney Disease (CKD) and Osteoporosis: Balancing Bone Health and Kidney Function

Chronic kidney disease (CKD) often coexists with osteoporosis, as impaired kidney function affects the body's ability to process and retain vital minerals, like calcium and phosphorus, crucial for bone health. CKD can also interfere with vitamin D production, decreasing bone density and an elevated fracture risk.

Managing osteoporosis alongside CKD requires close medical supervision to balance bone health with kidney function. A renal-friendly diet—low in phosphorus and sodium and adjusted for protein—can protect the kidneys while supporting bone health. Calcium supplementation should be approached cautiously, as excess calcium can burden the kidneys. Instead, foods that naturally support bone health, like leafy greens, bell peppers, and berries, are recommended.

It is crucial to work with a nephrologist to tailor a bone health plan that considers CKD limitations. Weight-bearing and low-impact exercises like walking and Tai Chi can support bone density without stressing the kidneys. Monitoring calcium, vitamin D, and phosphorus levels regularly helps tailor a balanced approach to managing CKD and osteoporosis.

Depression and Osteoporosis: Prioritizing Mental and Bone Health

Depression is linked to an increased risk of osteoporosis due to hormonal imbalances, lifestyle factors, and some antidepressants that may impact bone density. Individuals with depression often experience lower physical activity and may have difficulty adhering to bone-healthy diets, leading to bone loss over time.

Addressing both conditions requires a comprehensive approach that includes mental and physical health support. Regular exercise, such as walking, yoga, or swimming, has shown benefits for both bone health and mood improvement. Omega-3-rich foods, like salmon and walnuts, along with leafy greens and vitamin D, simultaneously support brain and bone health.

Counseling, cognitive behavioral therapy, and support groups can be invaluable for managing depression. Consulting with a psychiatrist familiar with bone health considerations can help adjust medications as needed. Small lifestyle adjustments, like a consistent sleep schedule and daily outdoor time, can improve mood and support vitamin D production, promoting a balanced approach to managing both depression and osteoporosis.

"No act of kindness, no matter how small, is ever wasted."

– Aesop

A Quick Favor to Pay It Forward

Dear Reader,

As our time together in these pages comes to a close, I have one small request—if the insights here have made a difference in your health journey, would you consider leaving a brief review?

Your words have incredible power:

- They help others struggling with similar challenges find this resource.
- They let me know what mattered most to you.
- They honor the healing journey we've shared

It only takes a minute:

1. Visit the book's Amazon page/Scan the QR code
2. Click "Leave a Review"
3. Share what helped you most (even just 2-3 sentences!)

From the bottom of my heart, thank you for letting me be part of your wellness story. Your voice makes this work worthwhile.

With gratitude,
Isabella

Conclusion

As we reach the end of our journey together, let's revisit the key points we've covered in this book. We've explored osteoporosis from multiple angles: understanding how it affects the body, looking at medical treatments, exploring natural remedies, and delving into practical ways to support and enhance bone health through diet, exercise, and emotional resilience. Along the way, we've also touched on the complex interplay between osteoporosis and other health conditions, recognizing how managing one area of health can directly benefit another.

One of the most important takeaways is that osteoporosis can be managed with the right knowledge and tools. Throughout this book, we've emphasized the value of staying informed, working closely with healthcare providers, and taking proactive measures. Knowing your bone density, identifying risk factors, and creating a tailored plan of action can make a powerful difference in how you live with osteoporosis.

Nutrition plays a fundamental role in maintaining bone health, and we've gone into detail about what to eat for optimal bone strength. A diet rich in calcium, vitamin D, and other essential nutrients forms the backbone of bone health. The recipes and meal plans provided offer ways to integrate these nutrients into your everyday routine, making healthy eating both enjoyable and effective. Remember, the choices you make in the kitchen can have a lasting impact on your bone strength and overall vitality.

Exercise has been another cornerstone of our discussion. Weight-bearing and muscle-strengthening activities are critical in supporting bone density and improving mobility. The exercises we've discussed range from simple weight-bearing moves to gentle balance practices, providing something for everyone, regardless of age or fitness level. Building a sustainable exercise routine that gradually increases in intensity can bolster your bones and keep you active.

The emotional and mental aspects of managing osteoporosis are equally important. We explored coping mechanisms, from building a strong support network to using mindfulness techniques that help manage stress. Emotional well-being, after all, is closely tied to physical health, and nurturing a positive outlook can make each step of this journey smoother and more fulfilling.

As you move forward, here's how to keep building on the foundation we've set in this book:

1. **Keep Learning and Stay Involved**
   Medical advancements continue to shape the landscape of osteoporosis care, and staying updated can empower you to make informed decisions. Whether it's a new diagnostic tool, a dietary recommendation, or a treatment option, staying engaged with credible sources and consulting with your healthcare provider ensures that you're always aware of the latest, most effective solutions.

2. **Take Action and Embrace Change**
   Small, consistent changes in diet, exercise, or routine can have a lasting positive impact. From making your home safer to incorporating bone-strengthening foods and exercises into your day, each step is a positive investment in your health. Explore the tips, tools, and resources shared in this book to craft a lifestyle that strengthens your bones and overall well-being.

3. **Stay Committed and Set New Goals**
   Managing osteoporosis is a lifelong commitment, but with dedication, it's entirely possible to lead a fulfilling, active life. Set milestones, celebrate each achievement, and adjust your goals as you progress. Persistence is key to maintaining bone health, building resilience, and enjoying a sense of accomplishment along the way.

This book aims to provide you with a thorough, compassionate guide to managing osteoporosis effectively. My mom's experience navigating this condition taught me a lot about resilience, the importance of being well-informed, and the power of small, deliberate actions. I share her story and what I've learned from it to support you in finding confidence and optimism in your own journey.

Thank you for allowing me to be part of your journey toward stronger bones and a vibrant, healthy life. Remember, you are never alone—there's a supportive community ready to help and encourage you. Stay positive, keep moving forward, and continue confidently embracing each step. You have the strength to meet osteoporosis's challenges head-on and create a life full of vitality and joy.

References

- *Global, regional prevalence, and risk factors ...*
  https://pubmed.ncbi.nlm.nih.gov/35687123/
- *Osteoporosis - Symptoms and causes - Mayo Clinic*
  https://www.mayoclinic.org/diseases-
  conditions/osteoporosis/symptoms-causes/syc-20351968
- *Osteopenia vs. osteoporosis: What is the difference?*
  https://www.medicalnewstoday.com/articles/osteopenia-vs-
  osteoporosis
- *Psychological state, quality of life, and body composition in ...*
  https://www.ncbi.nlm.nih.gov/pmc/articles/PMC2836755/
- *Osteoporosis - Symptoms and causes*
  https://www.mayoclinic.org/diseases-
  conditions/osteoporosis/symptoms-causes/syc-20351968
- *Bone density scan (DEXA scan) - How it is performed - NHS*
  https://www.nhs.uk/conditions/dexa-scan/what-happens/
- *T-Score Vs. Z-Score for Osteoporosis: What the Results Mean*
  https://www.healthline.com/health/t-score-vs-z-score-osteoporosis
- *Osteoporosis: An Update on Screening, Diagnosis ...*
  https://www.ncbi.nlm.nih.gov/pmc/articles/PMC10084730/
- *FDA approves new treatment for osteoporosis in postmenopausal
  women at high risk ...* https://www.fda.gov/news-events/press-
  announcements/fda-approves-new-treatment-osteoporosis-
  postmenopausal-women-high-risk-fracture
- *Adverse Effects of Bisphosphonates: Implications for ...*
  https://www.ncbi.nlm.nih.gov/pmc/articles/PMC2704135/
- *Role of Traditional Chinese Medicine in Bone ...*
  https://www.ncbi.nlm.nih.gov/pmc/articles/PMC9194098/
- *Calcium and vitamin D supplementation in osteoporosis*
  https://www.uptodate.com/contents/calcium-and-vitamin-d-
  supplementation-in-osteoporosis
- *New Insights into Nutrients for Bone Health and Disease*
  https://www.ncbi.nlm.nih.gov/pmc/articles/PMC10303436/

- *Top 15 Calcium-Rich Foods (Many Are Nondairy)*
  https://www.healthline.com/nutrition/15-calcium-rich-foods
- *Vitamin D for Good Bone Health - OrthoInfo - AAOS*
  https://orthoinfo.aaos.org/en/staying-healthy/vitamin-d-for-good-bone-health/
- *The Mediterranean Diet in Osteoporosis Prevention*
  https://www.ncbi.nlm.nih.gov/pmc/articles/PMC7915719/
- *Exercising with osteoporosis: Stay active the safe way*
  https://www.mayoclinic.org/diseases-conditions/osteoporosis/in-depth/osteoporosis/art-20044989
- *Exercising with osteoporosis: Stay active the safe way*
  https://www.mayoclinic.org/diseases-conditions/osteoporosis/in-depth/osteoporosis/art-20044989
- *Pilates for Osteoporosis: Safety, Benefits, and Risks*
  https://www.healthline.com/health/fitness/pilates-for-osteoporosis
- *Exercise for Your Bone Health | NIAMS*
  https://www.niams.nih.gov/health-topics/exercise-your-bone-health
- *What Are the Must-Have Home Modifications for Aging in Place*
  https://www.assistedliving.org/home-modifications-for-seniors-aging-in-place/
- *The Role of Assistive Devices in Preventing Falls at Home*
  https://www.vha.ca/blog/the-role-of-assistive-devices-in-preventing-falls-at-home/
- *Fear of Falling in Older Adults: A Scoping Review ...*
  https://www.ncbi.nlm.nih.gov/pmc/articles/PMC8629501/
- *Living with Osteoporosis: 8 Exercises to Strengthen Your ...*
  https://www.healthline.com/health/managing-osteoporosis/exercises-to-strengthen-your-bones
- *Emotional wellbeing and osteoporosis*
  https://theros.org.uk/information-and-support/osteoporosis/living-with-osteoporosis/everyday-life/emotional-wellbeing-and-osteoporosis/

- *Building a Strong Support System for Chronic Illness ...*
  https://www.lotusmedicalcentre.com.au/building-a-strong-support-system-for-chronic-illness-management/
- *Mental Health: How It Affects Your Physical Health*
  https://www.webmd.com/mental-health/how-does-mental-health-affect-physical-health
- *Living with Osteoporosis and Helping Others - Bone Talk*
  https://www.bonetalk.org/articles/one-mans-journey-living-with-osteoporosis-and-helping-others
- *Five latest advancements in osteoporosis research*
  https://www.labiotech.eu/best-biotech/osteoporosis-research/
- *Bone Health & Osteoporosis Foundation: Home*
  https://www.bonehealthandosteoporosis.org/
- *Efficacy of Osteoporosis Prevention Smartphone App on ...*
  https://www.ncbi.nlm.nih.gov/pmc/articles/PMC7105101/
- *About Clinical Trials*
  https://www.bonehealthandosteoporosis.org/patients/clinical-trials/about-clinical-trials/